S0-AZB-390

Publisher's Note

The editors of FC&A have taken careful measures to ensure the accuracy and usefulness of the information in this book. While every attempt has been made to assure accuracy, errors may occur. We advise readers to carefully review and understand the ideas and tips presented and to seek the advice of a qualified professional before attempting to use them. The publisher and editors disclaim all liability (including any injuries, damages, or losses) resulting from the use of the information in this book.

The health information in this book is for information only and is not intended to be a medical guide for self-treatment. It does not constitute medical advice and should not be construed as such or used in place of your doctor's medical advice.

Ordinary Ailments, Extraordinary Cures

By Frank K. Wood and the Editors of
FC&A Medical Publishing

"Beloved, I pray that in all respects you may
prosper and be in good health, just as your
soul prospers." – 3 John 1:12

FC&A
103 Clover Green
Peachtree City, GA 30269

Produced by the staff of FC&A
Distributed to the trade by National Book Network

ISBN 1-932470-01-8

Table of contents

Acne

Clearing up acne myths

Slumber parties, geometry, prom, summer camp – and acne. Manager meetings, car payments, PTA – and acne. You don't have to be a teenager to get hit with pimples and blackheads. A recent survey found that 81 percent of people with acne were 15 to 44 years old. If you find yourself over 30 and battling breakouts, don't despair. First, learn the truth behind acne myths – then form a plan of attack.

Myth #1: Acne will go away on its own. Some people think if you leave pimples alone, they will eventually go away. While it is true many breakouts will heal sooner or later, if you treat acne right away, you are less likely to suffer from both emotional and physical scarring.

If you're looking for a treatment without chemicals, try a natural antibacterial from Australia called tea tree oil. A 5-percent tea tree oil gel was tested against the popular acne treatment benzoyl peroxide lotion, and it came out a winner. The tea tree oil reduced breakouts just as effectively as the benzoyl peroxide but with fewer side effects. Look for tea tree oil lotion and soap at your local bath and body shop.

Myth #2: Acne is caused by dirt. Pimples form when oil from overactive oil glands mixes with dead skin cells and plugs up your pores. To keep your face clean, wash it twice a day with mild, unscented soap and warm water. Scrubbing your face constantly and using harsh soaps will not wash away your acne. In fact, it can make the condition worse.

Here's a natural cleanser you can easily make at home. Heat some lemon juice until barely warm and add two egg whites. Whip this mixture until it forms a thick paste. Store any unused cleanser in the refrigerator.

Myth #3: Acne is caused by the foods you eat. Although lots of healthy foods, like fresh fruits and vegetables, are important to healthy skin, eating chocolate and pizza will not cause acne. Just eat a balanced diet and drink lots of water.

Myth #4: Sunlight helps acne. Tanning or using a sunlamp on your face may hide your acne, but only temporarily. The long-term effects of sun exposure – aging and skin cancer – far outweigh any immediate benefits. Use a sunscreen, but choose one that's oil-free.

Myth #5: Squeezing pimples helps them heal faster. The exact opposite is true. You are much more likely to cause redness and swelling, even scarring, by picking. If you must do something, wrap an ice cube in a soft cloth and hold it to the blemish for a few minutes every hour.

Self-help for acne

Who needs expensive acne medications? Often, you can fight breakouts with everyday household items.

Mash acne with potatoes. Use potato power to fight your next acne breakout. Rub half a raw potato over your face, leave the juice on for 20 to 30 minutes, and rinse with cold water. Sound strange? Then consider this – when was the last time Mr. Potato Head had a pimple?

Keep an eye on your complexion. Pimples are a sight for sore eyes. But you can get rid of them with eye drops that relieve redness. Just squeeze a few drops onto a cotton swab and hold it against your pimple for about 30 seconds. Very soon you'll see a clear improvement.

Make haste – and paste. For clearer skin, combine two table-spoons of oatmeal and enough olive oil to make a paste. Massage the paste into the affected area, and leave it there for about five minutes. Then rinse with warm water.

Brew up a strong defense. Do you feel trouble brewing on your face? At the first sign of a pimple, smear a mixture of brewer's yeast and plain yogurt on your face. Leave it there for a few minutes before wiping it off.

Try this minty-fresh approach. Just dab a bit of toothpaste on your pimple at night. The next morning, wipe off the dried tooth-paste with a clean, warm washcloth, and the annoying redness will be gone.

Discover sour power. Try dabbing blemishes several times a day with lemon juice. Or lay a slice of lemon over your breakouts for a few minutes.

Here's how the experts treat acne

Most acne is caused by overactive oil glands in your face, upper back, and chest. If you decide to seek help from a dermatologist, he may prescribe one or more of these products, depending on the severity of your acne.

Peeling agents. These include lotions or ointments you apply in a thin film. They will dry your skin and often cause redness. If you suffer from mild acne, your dermatologist will most likely recommend starting with one of these products.

- Benzoyl peroxide (Benoxyl, Oxy 10) is available over-the-counter or in stronger doses through a prescription. It helps reduce acne-causing bacteria and unblocks clogged pores.

- Tretinoin, retinoic acid, or vitamin A acid (Renova, Retin-A) prevent pimples and blackheads from forming. They will make your skin very sensitive to sunlight. To reduce skin irritation, avoid using other drying lotions, medicated cleansers and make-up, or skin products containing alcohol.

■ Salicylic acid, sulfur, or resorcinol help remove dead skin cells. You'll find these ingredients in many popular over-the-counter acne products.

Topical antibiotics. These creams or ointments reduce the amount of bacteria on your skin or suppress the number of bacteria in your oil glands. You may use these alone or with other products, such as oral antibiotics.

They can cause redness, tingling, or stinging and often dry out your skin. Some topical antibiotics may seem to make your skin oilier. If you use them with other acne treatments or with soaps, cosmetics, or shaving products containing alcohol, your skin may become irritated. Topical antibiotics will make your skin more sensitive to the sun.

Some examples are azelaic acid cream, clindamycin phosphate, erythromycin, metronidazole, and tetracycline hydrochloride.

Oral medications. These drugs are prescribed for cases of acne that don't clear up with milder treatments. You can use these alone or along with topical products.

■ Tetracycline hydrochloride (Achromycin) is an antibiotic for moderate acne. This drug can make your skin very sensitive to the sun. Other antibiotics in the tetracycline family are doxycycline hydrochloride and minocycline hydrochloride.

■ Birth control pills are often prescribed for women with acne. They decrease the effects of male hormones, which stimulate oil glands.

■ Isotretinoin (Accutane) is prescribed for severe acne. It shrinks oil glands and changes the consistency of the oil produced, making it less likely to block your pores. Talk with your doctor about the possible side effects of isotretinoin. They include depression, headaches, fatigue, dry eyes and lips, extreme dry skin, and high cholesterol and triglyceride levels. This drug can also cause severe birth defects if taken during pregnancy.

Allergies

Take charge of annoying symptoms

If itchy eyes, a runny nose, sneezing, and coughing are part of your everyday life, you could be super sensitive to common substances, like plant pollen, dust mites, mold, animal dander, feathers, or chemicals. Normally harmless to most people, these allergens can cause the mucous membranes in your eyes, nose, throat, and sinuses to go wild.

Although there is no cure for allergies, you can control them by avoiding things that trigger your symptoms in the first place.

■ Choose nonaerosol household cleaning products.

■ Avoid cigarette and cigar smoke.

■ Keep the humidity inside your house at less than 50 percent to reduce mold.

■ Stay away from birds, cats, and dogs.

■ Plan your outdoor activities away from seasonal grasses and weeds that release pollen.

■ After working in your yard or garden, remove your clothes, shower, and rinse your nostrils with salt water.

■ Install a filter system on your air conditioner.

■ Dust with a wet cloth to trap allergens. A dry cloth simply scatters the dust.

■ Replace wall-to-wall carpeting with wood or vinyl floors. Put down area rugs that can be cleaned or washed regularly.

■ Repair leaking faucets or pipes to reduce the growth of mold.

And here's another thing you should consider – dust mites. These tiny insects live in bedding, rugs, carpets, cushions, stuffed toys, and mattresses. They eat dead, sloughed-off human skin cells and give off waste material that can trigger allergic reactions.

The good news is mites can be killed by hot-water washing or dry cleaning. This means fabric items more frequently washed or dry-cleaned are less likely to contain dust mites and other allergens.

Wool clothing and linens, for instance, usually contain more mites because they are washed less often. Remember, if you wash your bedding in cold water, you'll remove most of the mite waste materials but not the live mites.

Here are several unbeatable ways to kill dust mites and remove their allergens:

- Choose clothes and linens that can be washed regularly in very hot water.

- Store out-of-season clothes and linens under dry conditions. Mites need moisture to survive.

- Wash or dry-clean items that have been stored for a season.

- Tumble items in a hot dryer.

- Cover your mattress and pillows with plastic.

- Place items in a deep freeze for at least 24 hours.

Simple solutions to soothe an itch

It's easy to irritate your skin. Anything from the sun to toxic plants, dust mites, and other pests can cause allergic rashes, itching, and sores. Just don't rush out and pay a fortune for expensive creams and ointments. Now it's easy, and cheap, to treat these irritations. Try these natural remedies that won't rub your sensitive skin the wrong way.

Brew a healing pot. Just a few cups of oolong tea may let you say so long to itchy, scaly skin caused by a type of allergic disorder called dermatitis. In a clinical trial, drinking one liter (a little more than a quart) of this Chinese beverage every day improved symptoms within one or two weeks. At the end of a month, two-thirds of the people in the study reported relief. Experts believe oolong tea contains certain compounds that block allergic reactions.

Resurrect an ancient cure. Aloe vera may have been one of the key ingredients used to preserve ancient Egyptian mummies. But you don't have to wait hundreds of years for its skin-saving benefits. The soothing liquid found inside the plump leaves of the aloe vera plant relieves all kinds of skin problems. You can use it fresh or substitute one of the many aloe-based products you'll find at your favorite drugstore.

Aloe creams, gels, and lotions soothe itches, rashes, sunburn, and blisters. Apply aloe lip balm to ease painful cold sores, and drink aloe juice for mouth ulcers. Remember, these products vary in quality and strength. If you don't get results with one, try a different brand or go to the more dependable living plant.

Doctor it with dairy. The uncomfortable itching of poison oak or ivy can ruin the fun of a day outdoors, but you may find relief inside your refrigerator. Make a soothing milk compress by soaking a clean cloth – linen, gauze, and soft flannel are good choices – in cool, whole milk. Place it loosely on the affected area for 10 to 20 minutes every hour until your skin feels better. This works well with painful sunburn and other skin conditions, too.

Gather a bouquet of healing blooms. Pick some marigolds, also known as calendula, for a colorful posy or a tea to soothe irritated skin. Steep the flowers in water and place a tea-soaked cloth over your rash. You'll be amazed how much better you'll feel. In addition, use the calendula tea as a rinse for sores in your mouth. Calendula also comes in oils, creams, and ointments that help wounds heal fast.

Another flower, chamomile, contains its own healing ingredient. In European tests, chamomile cream was almost as effective as hydrocortisone in relieving some skin problems.

Apply a poultice. You may not know what a poultice is, but if you're suffering from a skin rash, you'll want to try one right away. This old-fashioned remedy is basically any warm, thick mixture of herbs, water, and other ingredients that you spread on your skin and cover with a cloth.

A witch hazel poultice can help dry up an oozing rash and relieve the pain. Stir five to 10 heaping teaspoons of finely chopped witch hazel leaves into a cup of water. Bring this to a boil and simmer for five to 10 minutes, then strain. Press the wet leaves against your rash and cover the area with a warm cloth to hold it in place. A poultice made from crushed flaxseeds mixed with hot water can also soothe and protect your irritated skin.

Say "nuts" to skin problems. Tannins in the leaves of the English walnut tree act as an astringent, tightening skin tissues and helping dry up any discharge. Boil five teaspoons chopped leaves in a cup of water. Strain this mixture and soak a soft cloth in the liquid. Apply the compress two to four times a day.

Another nutty solution to a variety of skin problems is almond oil. You'll often find it in commercial lotions and ointments that soften and soothe the skin. Experts consider almond oil safe, but if you have food allergies, consider a different treatment.

Soak your troubles away. A relaxing bath may be just the thing to relieve allergic symptoms – just leave out the bubbles and turn down the heat. Instead, mix some oatmeal, baking soda, or vinegar in a tub of cool water to ease the itching. For the discomforts of poison oak or ivy, also try spreading a thick paste of baking soda and water over the affected area.

Laugh off your rash. Humor may truly be the best medicine when it comes to allergies. Japanese researchers exposed people with a history of allergic reactions to various allergens. Welts appeared, but shrank in those who watched a classic Charlie Chaplin film. Welts stayed the same in those who watched a weather report instead. Find out what tickles your funny bone – it just might save your skin.

Alzheimer's disease

Stock your cupboards to slash your risk

"I have recently been told that I am one of the millions of Americans who will be afflicted with Alzheimer's disease," Ronald Reagan, former president of the United States, announced in November 1994. "I intend to live the remainder of the years God gives me on this Earth doing the things I have always done," he declared. "Unfortunately, as Alzhei-mer's disease progresses, the family often bears a heavy burden. I only wish there was some way I could spare Nancy from this painful experience."

In his message, Reagan summed up the tragedy of Alzheimer's disease (AD). Those suffering from AD face the reality of losing touch with their old lives. Family and friends are forced to watch a loved one slowly fall victim to the dreadful condition.

Scientists aren't sure exactly what's behind AD. Some suspect a certain gene — apolipoprotein E4 allele (Apo E4) — plays a major part in the brain's decline. Other experts believe years of oxidative stress also are at the root of the problem.

Whatever causes Alzheimer's disease attacks the part of your brain that controls speech, thoughts, and memory. You gradually lose the power to recall the past and the ability to carry out your daily life. AD usually hits around age 65 and older, and your risk goes up each year after that.

Through this dark cloud, there is a ray of hope. According to AD experts like Dr. Grace Petot, a professor at Case Western Reserve University, people can change their lifestyles to lower their risk. Boost your fruit and vegetable intake for a start. Petot discovered that many AD sufferers ate fewer fruits and veggies as adults.

Science, she suggests, also points to a connection between heart disease and Alzheimer's. So eating a heart-healthy diet might protect you, too. That means a diet based on high-fiber, low-fat foods. It's also a good idea to exercise both your mind and your muscles. "Keeping the brain active and the body active," Petot says, "is beneficial in many ways."

Make sure you're getting enough of these brain protectors in your diet to help you fight AD.

Antioxidants. Thanks to cutting-edge research, experts now hope AD can one day be prevented. Antioxidants, those powerful substances that fend off cancer and heart disease, might also safeguard your brain against free radicals. Antioxidants appear to slow – and even reverse – the memory loss caused by free-radical damage.

Supplements usually only contain one antioxidant, so eat a variety of fruits and vegetables to get the most benefits. Fruits and vegetables are rich in many antioxidants – not just beta carotene or vitamin C. They also contain natural plant chemicals called flavonoids, which act like antioxidants. Flavonoids make memory-saving marvels out of snacks like blueberries, strawberries, and spinach.

B vitamins. You also need foods rich in B vitamins to help protect your brain from AD. At least two studies show Alzhei-mer's sufferers have lower levels of folate and B12 than their peers who don't have AD. Low B-vitamin levels, according to several other studies, appear to lead to lower scores on IQ and memory tests.

Vitamin B12 helps your body make neurotransmitters, chemicals that help carry messages between your nerves and your brain. Another B vitamin, thiamin, helps nerve signals travel from your brain to different parts of your body. These important tasks could be why a lack of B vitamins can affect your brain's health.

To get more folate into your diet, try dark leafy greens, broccoli, beets, beans, and okra. Meats, eggs, and dairy products are good sources of B12. For older adults, who might have trouble absorbing

B12, experts suggest eating fortified breakfast cereals. Wheat germ, nuts, beans, and rice are good sources of thiamin.

Omega-3s. Look to the sea to find help against Alzheimer's. Fish are the greatest source of omega-3 fatty acids. These fat molecules protect against heart disease and inflammation and may lead the attack against Alzheimer's as well. One of AD's possible causes is beta-amyloid plaque, clumps of protein that build up in the victim's brain. Experts believe beta amyloid might be connected with inflammation of the brain's blood vessels. So it makes sense that anti-inflammatory omega-3 fatty acids could help.

Experts recommend eating at least two servings of salmon, tuna, mackerel, or other cold-water fish per week. For you landlubbers who think fish are for the birds, get your omega-3 from flaxseed, walnuts, and dark leafy greens. And while you punch up omega-3, limit your intake of omega-6 fatty acids. They compete with omega-3 and can cause inflammation. Foods high in omega-6 include fried and fast foods, salad dressings, and baked goods.

Calcium. Calcium already appears to fight breast and colon cancer, defeat digestion problems, help high blood pressure, and shore up fragile bones. Now add to that list prevent memory loss, senility, and forms of dementia like Alzheimer's. Calcium, experts say, plays a role in the way brain and nerve cells work together. So don't fall short. Include low-fat dairy products in your diet, drink orange juice fortified with calcium, and remember to eat beans and broccoli. If you are still concerned, talk with your doctor about taking calcium supplements.

6 ways to protect your brain

The calorie count of a diet soda is pretty attractive if you're watching your weight – it's zero. But the artificial sweetener that saves you all those calories may harm your brain in the long run. A new study shows that aspartame, the artificial sweetener in most diet drinks, may cause memory loss.

Students at Texas Christian University who regularly drank diet sodas with aspartame were more likely than those who didn't use aspartame to experience long-term memory problems, researchers found. While they did just as well as people who didn't use aspartame in laboratory memory tests, they were more likely to forget details of personal routines or whether they had completed a task.

This doesn't mean you have to ditch your diet drinks completely. Other studies on the effects of aspartame have had mixed results. But if you want to play it safe, perhaps you should switch to another no-calorie beverage – water. And while you're at it, follow these other simple steps to protect your memory and help keep Alzheimer's at bay.

Control blood pressure and cholesterol. New evidence shows high blood pressure and high cholesterol not only damage your heart, they could also harm your brain. That's why it's more important than ever to control those conditions by exercising, eating right, and getting regular checkups.

If you can't control your cholesterol and blood pressure naturally, you may have to take medication. Luckily, some heart-protecting drugs may also protect against Alzheimer's, giving you a double dose of defense. A recent study at Boston University School of Medicine found statin cholesterol medicines lowered risk of dementia by up to 70 percent. Another study found two particular types of statins – lovastatin and pravastatin – protected against AD, but a third – simvastatin – did not. Other types of cholesterol medicines also did not lower the risk of Alzheimer's, so if you're interested in this potential treatment, you need to discuss your medication with your doctor.

Reach for some aspirin. Doctors often recommend aspirin to help prevent heart disease. Now research finds regular use of aspirin may also help you avoid Alzheimer's. Other nonsteroidal anti-inflammatory drugs (NSAIDs) may put the brakes on this disease as well. One study found that the popular pain reliever ibuprofen lowered the risk of AD by 60 percent. These inexpensive remedies might be just what you need to stem the tide of Alzheimer's, but they can have serious side effects, like stomach irritation and bleeding. Talk with your doctor before starting any treatment.

Consider the benefits of estrogen. Estrogen replacement therapy (ERT) may do more than ease hot flashes – it could keep your mind sharper. Several studies have found ERT lowers your risk of developing Alzheimer's disease and other dementia.

It could even give your memory a boost right now. A recent study found that women on ERT performed better on tests of mental abilities. The results were supported by brain images showing estrogen users had more blood flow to the hippocampus, an area of the brain involved in memory formation.

But not all research supports estrogen as a way to fend off Alzheimer's. Two recent studies found ERT did not improve the mental abilities of women who already had the disease. And another study found that estrogen helped protect against Alzheimer's only in women with certain genes.

As usual, you need to look at all sides of the issue and talk with your doctor about whether ERT is right for you. But if you decide to take estrogen for other reasons, there's a chance your brain may benefit as well.

Build up your knowledge. An excellent way to protect your brain is to flex your mental muscle often. Every time you learn something, you establish new connections between brain cells, called synapses. Alzheimer's disease destroys synapses, but experts believe the more you have, the longer it takes AD to affect your mental abilities.

You don't have to go back to school to maintain your brain, either. Any kind of learning is useful, so take up a new hobby, work crossword puzzles, or read a variety of interesting books. Everything you learn builds a reserve of knowledge that may protect your brain from the ravages of Alzheimer's disease.

Make an effort to exercise. While you're building your brain, don't neglect your body. According to research, regular exercise not only improves your heart but your mind as well. A fit heart and clear arteries supply your brain with oxygen-filled blood. This helps guard against memory loss and Alzheimer's.

In one study, a group of seniors found that four months in an exercise routine – such as walking, running, or riding a stationary bike for 30 minutes every day, three days a week – improved their memory and problem-solving skills. And every step counts, according to a study of almost 6,000 women ages 65 and older. Every extra mile a week the women walked reduced their risk of mental decline by 13 percent.

Find time to socialize. Have fun and stimulate your brain at the same time by going out often with friends and family. Research finds that people who engage in lots of leisure activities, such as visiting with friends, doing volunteer work, and going to church, are much less likely to lose their mental abilities as they grow older.

Warning: 10 early signs of Alzheimer's

Every time you forget a name or lose your glasses, you may panic, thinking you have Alzheimer's. Chances are, you're perfectly fine. In fact, worrying about your memory loss is a good sign that you're OK. People with severe memory problems are usually unaware of their own lapses, so it may be up to family members to notice.

Unfortunately, a recent study found that one out of five families with a member who has mental problems was unable to recognize the problem. Detecting Alzheimer's early may help slow its progress, so look at this list of early warning signs that you or a loved one may have the disease.

Forgetfulness. The most well-known sign that you might have Alzheimer's is simply forgetfulness. While it's normal to forget names or lose your keys once in a while, frequent forgetfulness may be a red flag. The classic example is that it is normal to forget your keys, but if you can't remember what the keys are for, it's time to seek help.

Speech problems. Sometimes a word is on the tip of your tongue, but you just can't get it out. Everyone has that experience occasionally, but if you often have trouble with simple words, or your speech is difficult to understand, you may have a problem.

Misplacing things. Some people lose track of their keys or the TV remote almost every day. But finding lost items in a strange place, like keys in the microwave or books in the refrigerator, should be cause for concern.

Personality changes. Everyone goes through changes in their lives. Some people become more laid-back and relaxed as they age, while others seem to turn into grumpy old men and women. Alzheimer's can cause profound personality changes, making a calm, sweet person frightened, paranoid, or confused.

Loss of judgment. You may think young people show poor judgment in their choice of clothes, but if you can't judge what clothing is appropriate for you to wear, you may be the one with a problem. If you put your socks on your hands, or wear shorts when it's snowing, you have lost your ability to judge.

Loss of interest. Everyone can lose interest in a slow-paced movie, but when you aren't interested in the things that used to bring you pleasure, like hobbies, that's a little more serious.

Problems with familiar tasks. Busy people often are distracted and may forget to finish something they started. Someone with Alzheimer's might prepare a meal and not only forget to serve it, but not remember she even made it in the first place.

Mood swings. Although most people are moody sometimes, going from one extreme to the other rapidly for no apparent reason is cause for concern.

Disorientation. If you get lost in a strange city, no one would accuse you of having Alzheimer's. If you get lost in your own neighborhood, that's another story. Place or time disorientation is an early symptom of Alzheimer's. If you easily forget what day it is or how to get to a familiar place, see your doctor.

Trouble "adding it up." Maybe math was your worst subject in school. Still, if doing simple math problems suddenly becomes more difficult, you may have a problem yourself. Math requires abstract thinking, connecting symbols (numbers) with a meaning. Abstract thinking is one of the first skills you lose with Alzheimer's.

Raise your glass to lower your risk

A toast to good health! If your glass is filled with wine, your old age may be filled with memories. A recent study conducted in France found that drinking some wine may lower your risk of Alzheimer's disease.

The study found that among moderate drinkers (people who drank three to four glasses of wine a day), the incidence of Alzheimer's was about 1 percent. About 5 percent of the non-drinkers and mild drinkers developed the disease.

Although moderate alcohol intake may protect against AD, alcoholism contributes to dementia, so don't overdo it. Researchers say there is no reason to advise elderly people who do not drink to start indulging. Also, the people in the study drank only wine, not beer or other alcoholic beverages.

If you don't drink, you shouldn't start in hopes of avoiding Alzheimer's. But if you already drink wine, you may have more reason to toast your good health.

Anemia

Give iron-poor blood a boost

Residents of a small town in Georgia have long been in the practice of eating kaolin, a white clay substance found a foot or so beneath the surface of the earth. These peculiar eaters display a behavior called pica, a hunger for things that aren't normally considered food.

Bizarre eating habits, such as ice chewing and clay eating, often point to a common nutritional deficiency, like anemia. Nutritionists estimate that 20 percent of adult women and 3 percent of adult men are affected by this condition.

Iron-deficiency anemia can be caused by blood loss, problems with your body's absorption of iron, or not getting enough iron in your diet. If you have iron deficiency anemia, it's important for your doctor to find out why your iron is low. Recent studies show that low iron levels can lead to heart disease and even death, especially in older people.

Symptoms include fatigue, difficult breathing, weakness, headache, fainting spells, and depression. You also might notice a paleness to the color of your skin, nail beds, and lower eyelids. In its later stages, anemia can cause rapid pulse, irregular heart rate, and chest pains. Women may notice abnormal menstruation. Men can experience loss of sex drive and impotence.

If your anemia is caused by too little iron in your diet, here are some ways to boost your iron naturally.

Eat some meat. The best food for replacing iron is red meat, particularly organ meats such as calf liver and kidney. For lighter fare, you might try poultry or seafood. The type of iron found in meat, fish, and poultry is more easily absorbed into your body than other types of iron.

A good rule of thumb is – the darker the meat, the greater the iron content. Dark meats are also rich in vitamin B12 and zinc, important nutrients in preventing anemia.

Don't forget the peas and beans. Since the best natural source of iron is red meat, a strict vegetarian diet can lead to iron deficiency. But with all that fat and cholesterol, you might be shy about loading up on liver. A simple solution to this problem is to eat white poultry with legumes, such as peas or dry beans. Studies show that the animal protein in the poultry helps your body absorb iron from the veggies.

No meat? No problem. If you think you need meat to get your iron, think again. Iron that doesn't come from meat sources is usually less concentrated and less easily absorbed by your body, but it still helps the fight against anemia. Some good alternative sources are eggs, dairy products, grains, and legumes. Dried fruits, nuts, and blackstrap molasses are also good sources of iron.

Think green and leafy. One of the best ways to make sure you get the iron you need is by eating leafy greens. While green leafy vegetables don't contain much iron, they do contain a lot of folic acid and other nutrients. Folic acid plays a key role in helping your body absorb iron and the equally important vitamin B12. So don't forget the greens.

Drink some juice. Everyone loves a tall glass of orange juice, but did you know it can also chase away anemia? Vitamin C makes it easier for your body to absorb iron. It is so important, in fact, that a lack of vitamin C can sometimes cause anemia. Sweet red peppers, citrus fruits, and strawberries are good sources of vitamin C.

Round up some iron allies. Iron may be the key to keeping your blood cells up and running, but just getting enough iron won't do much good unless you eat a healthy diet. Vitamin A, vitamin E, thiamin (B1), riboflavin (B2), and copper are important ingredients for healthy blood. Foods rich in these vitamins and minerals help your body hold on to the iron it gets. Liver, dark green vegetables, and dairy products are great sources of riboflavin and vitamin A. Shellfish, nuts, cereals, and legumes are good providers of copper and thiamin, and for extra vitamin E, try some wheat germ.

Fire up the skillet. For an extra boost of iron in your diet, why not shut off the microwave and get out the pan? Research shows that foods cooked in cast-iron skillets are higher in iron.

Anxiety

How to live with stress

You don't need a doctor to tell you stress isn't healthy, but you may need help learning to deal with it.

When you're stressed, you can feel your heart pounding, your hands sweating, and your head throbbing. If your tension is ongoing – say you're the caretaker of a sick relative – you might experience a sense of anxiety that never quite leaves.

While all these sensations are certainly unpleasant, there's a darker, more dangerous side to stress.

- Heart disease. When you're under pressure, your heart takes a lot of abuse. The anxiety stress causes can lead to high blood pressure, atherosclerosis (hardening of your arteries), and abnormal heart rhythms.

- Sleep disturbances. You don't necessarily suffer from a sleep disorder or disease if you find yourself tossing and turning all night. Too much daily pressure can disrupt your internal clock. Insomnia caused by stress can be fixed – but not with sleeping pills.

- Weakened immune system. Constant stress can affect your ability to fight sickness and leave you vulnerable to disease. You also may recover from surgery and wounds more slowly. Some researchers think stress might even damage your body's ability to repair cells and lead to cancer.

- Prostatitis. Stressed-out men may suffer more from prostate disease than those who are relaxed. Anxiety triggers an increase in the hormone prolactin, which can cause prostate inflammation. On top of that, stress has been linked to high PSA (prostate-specific antigen), an indicator of increased prostate cancer risk.

■ Inflammatory bowel disease. Studies show that while stress may not cause digestive diseases, like Crohn's and ulcerative colitis, it can trigger attacks and make symptoms worse.

So now that you're motivated to reduce stress for your health's sake, here's how to do it.

Bite into breakfast. Your mother always said it was the most important meal of the day, and she was right. Researchers in England found that breakfast eaters – who tend to have healthier lifestyles overall – have more energy and feel less stressed than those who skip breakfast. And cereal eaters feel better regardless of their other health habits. So put some fuel in your tank before you start your day.

Don't skimp on sleep. No matter how much you have to do, get at least eight hours of shut-eye. If anxiety keeps you from drifting off, don't stay in bed worrying. Get up, experts say, and do something relaxing – watch some mindless TV or look through a magazine. If your brain keeps racing, make a list of what's bothering you and then let it go until tomorrow.

Take a vacation. You dream of getting away, but all your responsibilities make it seem impossible. That's exactly why you should go. A relaxing vacation won't just renew you for a week or two. Interviews revealed vacationers felt better physically up to five weeks after a get-away.

If you're a full-time caretaker, you need time off on a regular basis to renew yourself. Find a relative or nursing service that can cover for a few weekends a month and occasionally for longer breaks.

Put on your gardening gloves. There's something soothing about digging in the dirt. Maybe it reminds you of days in the sandbox, or perhaps it just brings you closer to nature. However it works, gardening not only rewards you with a prettier yard, it also lets you get rid of some of those worries along with the weeds.

Karin Fleming, HTR, president of The American Horticultural Therapy Association, says, "Gardening is a great all-around exercise that can be enjoyed by people of all ages and abilities. It helps tone muscles, which promotes healthy bones, and it helps maintain flexibility, stamina, and strength. It is also a known fact that gardening helps reduce stress and lower blood pressure."

Laugh at life. You might not see anything funny about your hectic schedule, but try to find the humor in each situation – it will give you the opportunity to relieve a little tension. Experts say people who can laugh at difficulties deal better with stress and, as a result, suffer fewer health problems. Even renting a funny movie can help. So start tuning in to the comedy around you. Instead of feeling as if life is out of control, you might start enjoying the show.

Forgive and forget. Holding a grudge is like holding yourself hostage. Anger and resentment can keep you from enjoying the good things in your life. When a group of men and women took a six-session course on forgiving others, they had fewer episodes of stress-related health problems. The health benefits of forgiveness were still obvious four months later at a follow-up session.

Massage your muscles. If you're keyed up, your muscles can feel tense and sore. A massage loosens those knots and helps you unwind and sleep better. Indulge.

Relax to music. Like taking a mini-vacation, listening to peaceful music can calm your nerves and ease muscle tension. Individual tastes will vary, but experts suggest giving classical music a try.

Write about it. Put your worries down on paper, and you might feel more in control of the situation. Some people believe keeping a journal helps them sort things out and identify possible solutions.

Get some sun. A sunny day can brighten your mood, but only if you get outside. Walk to the mailbox or a friend's house and the sunlight will boost your melatonin, a hormone that buffers the effects of stress and can help you sleep better.

Pray. If you believe in the power of prayer, you're not alone. In fact, for stress management and a general sense of well-being, seniors use prayer more than any other alternative treatment. You'll also be glad to know having others pray for your health, even if you don't know about it, could speed your recovery. And if you're a caregiver, praying may help increase your ability to cope with stress.

Confide in a counselor. Sometimes you just need someone to help you sort things out. Counseling is a great way to get some expert advice when anxiety and stress feel overwhelming. Chances are good that your health insurance will cover it. Ask your doctor for a referral or confide in a trusted minister, priest, or rabbi. Either way, you'll feel better after talking with someone who cares.

Get a lift with aromatherapy

The research is out, and the verdict is in – aromatherapy can relieve tension and daily stress. To lift your spirits and calm your mind, experiment with these essential oils – bergamot, cedarwood, frankincense, geranium, hyssop, lavender, sandalwood, orange, and ylang ylang.

Just remember, never place undiluted essential oils directly on your skin or in your mouth. Instead dilute them in "carrier oils," like almond, apricot, jojoba, and grapeseed oils.

◆ For the perfect massage, add 10 to 20 drops of essential oil to every 1 ounce of carrier oil.

◆ Get a steamy bath going and add five to 10 drops of essential oil and 1 ounce of carrier oil. Soak for at least 15 minutes to help you relax.

◆ Dab a handkerchief with three to four drops of your favorite oil. Whenever and wherever stress strikes, sniff it at arm's length for instant relief.

◆ For a stress headache, soak a hand towel in a mixture of a half-cup of water and five to 10 drops of oil. Hold the compress to your forehead until the towel is cold.

◆ A 10-minute footbath with hot water and a few drops of essential oil, especially lavender, will make you feel pampered and peaceful.

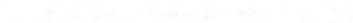

Banish stress with better breathing

In a hurry? Under pressure? Worries got you feeling low? Just slow down, relax, and take a deep breath. Simple, but very good, advice. Under stress, most people tend to breathe high up in their chests, taking short, shallow, rapid breaths.

This is appropriate in times of physical danger. It's part of the "fight or flight" response you inherited from your cave-dwelling ancestors. If you need to get out of the way of a speeding car, for example, it gets you moving before you have time to think about it.

But when dealing with stresses brought on by your job or problems in your family, running away from them or fighting would only make things worse. Slower, deeper breathing can help you settle down. And once you are calm and relaxed, you can think first, then act more sensibly.

Psychologist and breathing expert Dr. Gay Hendricks is an advocate for what he calls "conscious breathing." In his book *Conscious Breathing: Breathwork for Health, Stress Release, and Personal Mastery*, you learn how to use your breath to relieve stress, handle emotions, increase energy, and improve your health. "We can consciously take deeper, slower breaths, and we can consciously shift our breathing from chest to belly," says Hendricks. "I have seen this simple but powerful piece of information change many lives."

Breathe out negative emotions. Hendricks finds breathwork especially helpful when dealing with the "big three" emotions – fear, anger, and sadness. He says when you first feel an emotion, if you pay attention, you'll notice a change in your breathing. This awareness is your first step in dealing with what you are feeling.

And, he says, when you are ready to let go of an emotion, using your breath is the fastest way. Notice where you feel the emotion in your body. With anger, for example, you may feel stress in your jaw and neck muscles. Focus your attention on those places. And as you inhale, imagine you are breathing into the tension there. As you exhale, let yourself feel it move out of your body.

"Many times that's all it takes," says Hendricks. "I have witnessed this done a thousand times now, but it still moves me to see the look on people's faces when they learn that they are the masters of their feelings."

Bring the zest back to your life. Stress can really zap your energy. In his practice, Hendricks sees a lot of people with chronic fatigue syndrome. He helps them use their breath to regain their vitality. "One great benefit of conscious breathing," he says, "is that it has a direct effect on energy level. Put simply, if you breathe effectively you have much more physical energy."

Research shows slow, deep breathing can be helpful not only for stress but for problems with blood pressure, asthma, or congestive heart failure. Here are some tips to help you make the most of your natural breathing ability.

- Breathe through your nose. Along with air, you also breathe in dust and other irritants. Your nose is designed to filter out these pollutants as well as to moisten and warm the air before it reaches your lungs. Although you may have to breathe through your mouth sometimes, your nostrils are the best passageway.

- Take it slow. Men generally breathe 12 to 14 times a minute, women 14 to 15 times a minute. Health experts tend to consider anything over 15 to be a signal of stress. According to Hendricks, with conscious breathing the rate of respiration usually slows to about 8 to 12 breaths per minute. With fewer breaths, your lungs don't have to work as much. Your heart rate will slow as well because it doesn't have to pump so hard to get oxygen throughout your body.

■ Go deep. While most people breathe high in the chest, Hendricks recommends breathing into the belly. This doesn't mean you actually breathe air into your stomach. As you pull the air deeper into your lungs, the diaphragm drops and pushes your abdomen out as if it were filled with air. With deep breathing, the air reaches the lower area of your lungs where more blood is available to carry healthy oxygen to your organs.

■ Empty your lungs fully. When you exhale, pull your abdomen in tightly to squeeze out all the old air. Then you'll have more room for plenty of fresh air on the next inhalation.

■ Stay in your comfort zone. Don't push yourself to breathe so deeply or hold your breath so long that it's unpleasant. It should be restful, not distressing. With practice, you'll gradually get comfortable with longer, deeper breaths.

Hendricks believes that breathing will play a major role in both medicine and psychotherapy in the 21st century. Conscious breathing is within everyone's control and is easy to learn. Make it a part of your daily life, and you'll be on your way to a more relaxed, stress-free existence.

Asthma

Breathe easier with exercise

Asthma may make exercise extra challenging, but definitely not impossible. Many people with asthma avoid exercise because they fear an exercise-induced asthma attack.

But you don't have to miss out on good health and good times. In the 1984 and 1988 Olympics, 120 of the U.S. athletes had asthma. And those athletes won 57 Olympic medals.

Exercise-induced asthma is extremely common, but, fortunately, it can be prevented and controlled. Follow these suggestions, and you'll be able to enjoy a fun, daily exercise program.

Choose an asthma friendly exercise. Some activities are easier on your lungs than others. Most experts believe exercise-induced asthma occurs when your lungs lose heat and water. There are three reasons for this – long periods of hard breathing, breathing in allergens, and breathing in cold air.

Therefore, sports such as running and bicycling, especially during the winter, will increase your chances of an exercise-induced attack. Long-lasting endurance sports, such as baseball and down-hill skiing, are less likely to trigger asthma than a high-intensity sport like basketball or soccer.

Water sports cause the least problems because the moist, warm air prevents the airways from cooling. Plus, walking and weight training rarely trigger asthma.

The key to maintaining an exercise program is to choose an activity you enjoy. It's a good idea to experiment with different sports until you find your niche.

Pick the proper environment. Try to exercise in warm, humid, unpolluted environments.

Bundle up. On cold days, wear a face mask or scarf over your nose and mouth. This will make the air you breathe warmer and more humid. Foam nylon masks will help warm the air before it enters your lungs.

Remember to inhale. Use an inhaler five minutes to an hour before vigorous exercise. Always carry your inhaler in case you need it during exercise as well.

Warm up and cool down. Always warm up thoroughly before starting vigorous exercise. Follow up with a long cool down after exercise. This is an excellent way to gradually increase your physical strength and lung capacity without triggering an asthma attack.

Follow a pre-exercise routine. Some athletes with asthma follow this routine – they use their inhaler, do five to 10 minutes of vigorous exercise, then completely cool down. Then they start playing their sport. This routine gives them a two-hour period during which they can exercise without suffering any asthma symptoms.

Watch what you eat. Avoid eating certain foods up to two hours before exercise. Shrimp, celery, peanuts, egg whites, almonds and bananas are some of the foods that can trigger exercise-induced attacks. Eating these foods before exercise can actually cause breathlessness, a drop in blood pressure, and extreme weakness.

Breathe through your nose. This will warm and moisten the air in your nasal passages. *Asthma and Exercise* by Nancy Hogstead and Gerald Couzens and *The Breath Approach to Whole Life Fitness* by Ian Jackson outline breathing techniques that will reduce your chances of an asthma attack during exercise.

Keep a positive attitude and believe in yourself. Don't give up exercise if you have a bad experience. One negative experience does not even compare to all of the positive benefits of exercise.

Finally, don't overdo it! Too much exercise isn't healthy for anyone. Fatigue, anemia, and the rapid deterioration of muscles are just a few of the adverse effects of too much exercise.

Asthma does not have to slow you down. A consistent exercise program will actually improve your asthma. You'll be able to play your favorite sports, have fun, and compete with the best of them.

11 secrets to avoiding attacks

Watch out for acetaminophen. Glutathione, an antioxidant found naturally in your lungs, is thought to prevent your trachea and bronchial tubes from becoming inflamed during an asthma attack. Acetaminophen (Tylenol) uses up this antioxidant, leaving your airways more vulnerable. Research shows a link between people who take acetaminophen frequently —weekly to daily — and severe cases of asthma. If you suffer from asthma and take acetaminophen regularly, talk with your doctor and follow his advice.

Stay away from sulfites. In an Australian study, about one-third of the asthma sufferers reported that alcohol, most frequently wine, triggered their asthma attacks. Experts say it's likely the sulfites in wine and other foods are the cause.

Sulfites preserve food and sterilize the bottles used for alcoholic beverages, like wine. Foods high in sulfites are dried fruits, except dark raisins and prunes; bottled lemon and lime juice; beer, wine, and wine coolers; pickled foods; molasses; dried potatoes; sparkling grape juice; wine vinegar; gravy; and maraschino cherries. You'll often find sulfite-treated foods in a salad bar. To avoid sulfites, read food labels in the store and ask at restaurants.

Consider caffeine. Caffeine can help relieve some asthma attacks by relaxing and expanding the air passages in your lungs — but don't overdo it. Too much caffeine can increase your blood pressure and heart rate and cause insomnia. A moderate amount, especially during an asthma attack, may feel like a breath of fresh air.

Defend yourself with fish oil. A study of Eskimo, Japanese, and Dutch populations links a diet high in omega-3 fatty acids, found in fish oil, to low instances of asthma. Small amounts of fish oil over a long period of time seem to give the best results. Good natural sources are mackerel, salmon, striped bass, lake trout, herring, lake whitefish, anchovy, bluefish, and halibut. If you'd like to try fish oil supplements, talk with your doctor first.

Just the thought of stepping into a cold bath may take your breath away. But if you are bothered by the wheezing and chest-squeezing feelings of asthma attacks, you can take comfort from an icy dip.

Research shows cold water baths can improve breathing — but don't stay in there too long. A quick bath in cold water for only one minute or a 30-second cold shower every day showed the greatest results.

So turn on the cold water, brace yourself, and jump in — and enjoy easy breathing.

Boycott processed foods. Much of the food you eat is processed. This means flavorings, preservatives, sweeteners, conditioners, and artificial colors are added to make the products look or taste better and last longer on the shelf. Amazingly, very few people react to the more than 2,000 FDA-approved additives routinely used in food, but there are exceptions. Some people will have an asthma attack after eating food artificially colored with FD&C yellow No. 5. It's used in cake mixes, chewing gum, ice cream, cheese, and soft drinks.

Mind your MSG. Many people think a flavor enhancer called monosodium glutamate (MSG) can bring on severe asthma attacks in people sensitive to this additive. For many years, Chinese food received most of the blame for the MSG reaction.

Now, it may be safe to order your favorite Chinese food. Several studies pointing the finger at MSG turned out to be flawed. The trouble was traced to heartburn, anxiety, depression, or other food allergies. Check with your doctor to be sure.

Breathe easier with ginkgo. Ginkgo may prevent broncho-spasms, a sudden narrowing of the main air passages from the windpipe to the lungs. If you have asthma, a bronchospasm feels like a tightening or squeezing in your chest that makes it difficult to breathe. Ginkgo biloba extract, or GBE, is sold as a food supple-ment. While no serious side effects have been reported, some peo-ple taking ginkgo experience headaches or digestive problems.

Knock off extra pounds. Your weight has a lot to do with how well you breathe. If you have asthma and are clinically obese, los-ing weight can improve your lung function, decrease your asthma symptoms, and restore your overall health. You may even be able to reduce your medication with your doctor's approval.

Heal your heartburn. You probably never thought heartburn could make it hard to breathe, but researchers have discovered a link between gastroesophageal reflux disease (GERD) and asthma. Studies show up to 80 percent of asthma sufferers also have GERD, a condition where stomach acid backs up into the esopha-gus, causing heartburn. If your breathing problems didn't start until you were an adult and there's no family history of asthma, heartburn could be causing your symptoms. Other signs are wheezing or coughing at night or after exercise or meals. If you treat your reflux disorder, you may find asthma relief, too.

Give up the gas. If you're cooking with gas, you're twice as likely to develop breathing problems – especially the wheezing and shortness of breath associated with asthma. If you already suffer from asthma, you could be making it worse. Nitrogen dioxide released from gas stoves can irritate respiratory tracts, especially in women, increasing their risk of asthma and serious asthma attacks. Using an exhaust fan doesn't seem to help since it only removes cooking odors and water vapor, not fumes.

Get out the vacuum. You may hate to do it, but vacuuming every week will help you breathe easier. Studies show there is a big dif-ference in the amount of allergens in a home vacuumed weekly as opposed to monthly.

Athlete's foot

Do-it-yourself tips for healthier feet

Joining a gym was a great idea, you tell yourself. You can stop by on the way home from work and squeeze in a workout before dinner. But one morning, you wake up and there's a red rash between your toes that itches like crazy. That's athlete's foot. It's the most common fungal infection in people, and about 10 percent of the population is scratching away at any one time.

The ailment got its name because "a lot of people, when they go into the gym or work out, they don't dry their feet off completely," says Dr. Chet Evans, dean of the School of Podiatric Medicine at Barry University in Miami, one of the nation's seven colleges of podiatric medicine. "They slip their socks on when their feet are still wet."

While the gym floor environment makes weekend warriors especially at risk for athlete's foot, the fungus can grow in any warm, dark, moist place, like your bathroom, says Dr. Bryant Stamford, director of the Health Promotion and Wellness Center and professor of allied health, School of Medicine, University of Louisville, Louisville, Ky.

You also increase your chances of athlete's foot by simply wearing shoes, especially without socks, wearing the same pair of shoes all the time, or forgetting to wash your socks often enough. If you'd leave it alone, the fungus itself would be very irritating, but it wouldn't be dangerous.

Fortunately, the fungus stays on the top layer of your skin, a layer that acts as your body's natural Band-Aid to keep invaders out. Once you scratch off that shield, you put yourself at risk for a more serious infection.

"That's the potential," Evans says, "especially if you're a diabetic, have impaired circulation, if you have an immune system depression, such as AIDS, or you're on medication for cancer therapy."

Try Epsom salt soaks. When you have athlete's foot, try soaking your feet in Epsom salt, 10 to 15 minutes, three times a day for three to five days. You can also soak your feet in a gallon of warm water with two capfuls of bleach. After soaking, make sure you dry your feet completely.

After your bath, take a cotton ball and dry your feet with rubbing alcohol. "It burns like a son of a gun, but it's a good antiseptic and dries out the area," Evans says.

Sprinkle with cornstarch. You can sprinkle some cornstarch on your feet to help keep them dry when you have athlete's foot, but Evans warns against using baking soda or talcum powder if the infection is weeping. That can create a crust and allow the fungus and other bacteria to spread underneath.

Keep it clean and dry. The easiest way to prevent athlete's foot is to keep your feet clean and dry, wash your feet with soap and water, and change your socks. You can use a foot powder, but make sure it's medicated, Evans says. Talcum powder smells nice, but that's about it. It won't kill the organisms on your feet.

Soak your feet in warm tea. If your feet sweat profusely, try putting a couple of tea bags in hot water just long enough to turn the water brown. Let it cool until it's warm and soak your feet for five to 10 minutes.

Tea contains tannins, natural chemicals that help pull excess moisture from your feet. A solution of one part vinegar to 10 parts water also works well. Dry your feet thoroughly after soaking. You also can spray your feet with an antiperspirant deodorant spray.

If your case of athlete's foot lasts for more than five to seven days, or seems to be affecting a toenail, see your doctor.

Back pain

Plan ahead to sidestep pain

Most people take their backs for granted until something goes wrong. Don't wait to become one of the 80 percent of people affected by back problems. Start babying your back today to avoid back problems tomorrow.

Watch out for bad posture. Practice good posture all the time – keep your back straight, not arched, and your shoulders level. Don't slump even when you're relaxing. If you have to stand for long periods, rest one foot on a low stool and shift your weight often. Wear comfortable shoes with good support and low heels. Change positions frequently, no matter what you're doing.

Sit up straight. Choose a chair that gives your lower back good support. Add a small cushion or rolled up towel to the small of your back, even when you're driving. Sit properly with both feet on the floor or on a low stool, and keep your hips and legs at a 90-degree angle. Keep your chair close enough to your desk so you don't have to lean forward. If you spend a lot of time sitting, get up now and then to stretch.

Practice safe lifting. Keep your spine straight. Either squat, bending your knees, or bend at the hips, not the waist. Use your arms and legs to lift and keep the object close to your body.

Enjoy restful sleep. If you like to sleep on your back, put a pillow under your knees. If you prefer sleeping on your side, keep your knees bent.

Get some exercise. A simple exercise program, combining aerobic, flexibility, and strengthening exercises, will help keep your back in good shape. Try to exercise for at least 30 minutes every other day. And remember to check with your doctor before starting an exercise program.

Stop smoking. Smoking is linked to many back disorders. Researchers say smoking makes bones weaker by slowing the production of new bone cells. Weak bones can cause back pain.

Maintain a healthy weight. If you're overweight, lose those extra pounds. They are putting extra pressure on your spine.

Best ways to soothe an aching back

Back pain is often a sign of a serious condition, but if you're sure you don't have a medical problem that needs professional attention, your discomfort is probably from overdoing it. First of all, stop doing whatever caused the attack. Don't try to work through the pain. Being tough won't win you any trophies. Then try these pain-relieving tips, and you'll be back in the swing of things before you know it.

Grab a pill and a pillow. Taking aspirin or ibuprofen is a quick way to stop the pain. These over-the-counter painkillers not only attack the discomfort, they also have anti-inflammatory power to help shrink swollen, inflamed muscles. Relax by lying on your back with a pillow under your knees or on your side with a pillow between your knees.

Cool it or warm it. An ice pack and a gentle back massage may help cool your searing pain. Here's a simple kitchen remedy that will combine the two. Fill a small paper cup with water and freeze it solid. Have your spouse or a friend tear the paper off one end of the cup, then use the ice to massage your aching muscles. Try to hang in there for about 10 minutes, repeating as often as once an hour. If heat soothes you better, treat your back to a warm heating pad. Just be sure to turn it off before you fall asleep.

Get some rest — then get going. A day of bed rest may be needed and deserved when your back is really hurting, but don't overstay your welcome. A recent study showed that back-pain sufferers who went about their daily activities got well faster than those who exercised or stayed in bed. Get up as soon as you feel like it, even for short periods. Resume your normal activities, but take things easy for a while. Save that tennis match for later when your body can bounce back as easily as the ball.

Bad breath

Fresh solutions for sweeter breath

Almost everyone has suffered from bad breath from time to time.
When you eat, pieces of food get caught between your teeth and
on your tongue. They break down and give off foul-smelling gases,
like hydrogen sulphide.

Although bad breath can be embarrassing, it's easy to fix. These
tips should help freshen your breath. If they don't, your bad breath
may be a sign of illness you shouldn't ignore.

Keep your mouth clean. Brush your teeth with a soft toothbrush
and fluoride toothpaste at least twice a day. Brush well along the
gumline and over all tooth surfaces. To remove food and plaque
from between your teeth, floss every day. Curve the floss around
each tooth to cover the side surfaces.

Don't forget to clean your tongue. It's a huge source of bacteria
and odor. If brushing your tongue is uncomfortable, use a special
tongue scraper or the side of a spoon to gently scrape that sticky,
germy film off your tongue. Either way, be gentle.

Soak your dentures. Dentures are a common source of bacteria
and bad breath. If you have removable dentures, braces, or plates,
keep them squeaky clean. Remove and brush them each night, and
soak them in a disinfectant solution. Your dentist can tell you the
best kind to use.

Beware of mouthwash. Antiseptic and deodorant mouthwashes
only cover up breath odor temporarily – for about 10 minutes to
an hour at most. Mouthwashes containing alcohol can throw off
your mouth's natural chemical balance and dry it out, which can
cause bad breath.

These homemade mouthwashes may improve your breath without drying out your mouth:

- Mix some Listerine or Cepacol and olive oil. Gargle and spit out three times a day.

- Rinse with a mixture of half hydrogen peroxide and half water (don't gargle).

Prescription mouthwashes containing chlorhexidine seem to be effective in preventing gum disease. In studies, this germ-killing mouth rinse reduced bacteria by 50 percent. If you aren't able to brush and floss properly because of a physical disability, this rinse may help you avoid dental problems.

See your dentist. Get regular dental exams and talk with your dentist about any problems you're having, like ill-fitting crowns. Twice-yearly checkups and cleanings will help keep your mouth healthy and sweet-smelling. If you have tooth decay or gum disease, both causes of bad breath, your dentist can fix the problem.

Shy away from certain foods. A spicy lunch, such as garlic chicken, liver and onions, fish, or a pastrami sandwich, can give you "death breath" by afternoon. But did you know eating meat makes your breath more pungent than eating fruits and vegetables?

Once the chemical compounds in certain foods get into your bloodstream, your lungs excrete the odor. Breath sprays or mints won't cover it up. Alcohol, coffee, and tobacco (either smoked or chewed) are also causes of bad breath.

Serve up nutritious meals. Eat lots of fresh fruits, vegetables, and whole grains, rather than foods loaded with sugar and fat. And don't forget calcium – it helps build strong teeth. Skim milk and other low-fat dairy foods are good sources. Broccoli, cabbage, cauliflower, beans, and nuts are also high in calcium. Eating yogurt or drinking buttermilk that contains active cultures will also douse bad breath. The active lactobacillus bacteria make it hard for other odor-causing bacteria to grow.

You can halt "hunger breath" by not skipping meals. If you skip meals, diet, or fast, you aren't supplying your body with enough nutrients, and it will begin to break down your internal supply of protein for energy. This process creates an odor you exhale from your lungs.

Drink lots of water. Saliva constantly washes anything out of your mouth that can cause bad breath. As you get older, your salivary glands produce less saliva. If your mouth is too dry, it generally gives off a bad odor. Be sure to drink lots of water, at least six to eight glasses a day, but don't constantly rinse your mouth. You may be washing away any saliva that will help fight bad breath.

Suck on hard candies, especially lemon drops. Eat lots of oranges, grapefruit, and other citrus fruits. To stimulate the flow of saliva naturally, eat high-fiber foods, like celery, and chew sugarless gum or parsley.

Dry mouth can also be caused by sinus or throat infections, exercise, stress, mouth-breathing, talking, and certain medications, like antihistamines, antidepressants, and anticoagulants.

Body odor

Tricks to tame offensive odor

Long, long ago, humans could sweat, go through hormone changes, and not bathe for weeks, and nobody minded the smell. In fact, this pungent scent was one of the ways we attracted the opposite sex.

Today, research shows that the way you smell matters more to the people around you than any other physical aspect, including the way you look. But that doesn't mean your wife will think your sweaty odor after you mow the lawn on a hot summer day is sexy.

With the arrival of running water, deodorant soaps, and chemical antiperspirants, things have changed. Most people can take care of body odor with a daily bath, antiperspirants, deodorants, and clean clothes. If you practice good hygiene and you're still not happy with the way you smell, you may be ready for stronger measures.

First, get feedback from a friend. Do you really smell bad, or do you just think you do? Some people's noses "hallucinate." It doesn't mean you're crazy. It just means you think you're smelling something that's not actually there.

Next, ask your doctor about your odor. Body odor can be a side effect of a drug you're taking or a sign of a serious disease. If bacteria or a fungus is causing your body odor, your doctor may be able to prescribe antibiotics to help you.

Take a look at your diet. Garlic and onions are the biggest food offenders. The smell can drift from your skin hours after you've eaten them. Some people smell fishy when they eat eggs, fish, liver, and beans. These foods are high in choline, which produces a substance called trimethylamine. Some people can't metabolize this substance properly, so they give off a funny smell when they eat certain foods.

Try some natural astringents. The author of the book *30-Day Body Purification* suggests bathing or rubbing your skin with certain herbs, which work to close the pores. These natural astringents are witch hazel, arnica lotion, calendula, and coriander extract. These herbs may also fight odor-producing bacteria.

Find odor-fighters in your kitchen. Dabbing lemon juice under your armpits or powdering with cornstarch or baking soda can absorb some odors.

Powder away foot odor. Having problems with foot odor? Dust your feet with cornstarch each morning before putting on your socks. Change socks and powder your feet again midway through the day.

Mind your minerals. Some people have improved the way they smell with mineral supplements. Make sure your daily multivitamin contains calcium, magnesium, and zinc.

Breast cancer

How to protect yourself

The statistics are enough to send cold chills down your spine. One in nine American women will develop breast cancer. So you wonder, does that mean for every group of nine women, one will be stricken with breast cancer?

Only if the nine women are randomly selected and have their entire lives ahead of them, which means newborn babies. Your risk as an older woman is actually much lower. For example, during your 50s, your chances of getting breast cancer are approximately 1 in 30 because you have already survived several decades of risk. While you are right to be concerned with the figures, don't overestimate the danger.

Know your family history. It wasn't too long ago that breast cancer was a taboo subject, not fit for polite conversation. Luckily, things have changed. If your extended family doesn't talk about such things, start asking questions. You have a right to know if other relatives have had breast cancer. If they have, it doesn't mean you will definitely get the disease, but you are at increased risk – especially if the relative is your mother, sister, or daughter. Knowing your family history can help you stay alert to symptoms and take prevention seriously.

Don't fear fibrocystic breast disease. At one time, experts thought this disease of fluid-filled cysts in breast tissue increased your chances of cancer. Now they believe there is no connection. But if your doctor says you have a proliferative breast disease, your risk is somewhat higher.

Ignore the rumor of the week. It's bad enough how fast rumors can spread by word of mouth, but now rumors can instantly reach millions by way of the Internet. Have you heard antiperspirants cause breast cancer? Not true. Neither is the one about mammograms causing cancer. Base your beliefs on facts supported by science, and leave the rumors to the tabloids.

Practice prevention. Instead of worrying – which won't protect you – take the following measures that could.

■ Monthly self-exam. Ask your doctor to show you how to do a self-exam. Check your breasts the week after your period or, if you're past menopause, the first of every month. Do the exam faithfully, and call your doctor if you find any unusual changes in skin texture, color, or shape. Also, watch for any swelling, pain, or discharge from a nipple. And, of course, report any suspicious lump or thickening of breast tissue.

■ Yearly mammogram at 40. Mammograms can be a little uncomfortable, but here's a statistic that makes the discomfort more than worth it. Your chances of surviving breast cancer jump to 95 percent with early detection. These radiographic pictures can find tiny changes in your breasts that you might not notice for several more years.

■ Healthy diet. Experts think you can reduce your risk up to 50 percent by eating plenty of fruits, whole grains, and vegetables and by going easy on fats and sweets. Maintaining a healthy body weight, especially after menopause, will also increase the odds in your favor.

■ Limit alcohol. One drink a day is the maximum you should allow yourself if you're serious about avoiding breast cancer. If the disease runs in your family, you should consider not drinking alcohol at all.

■ Exercise. After checking with your doctor, add some sort of workout to your daily routine – even walking will do– and aim for 45 minutes to an hour. Choose something you enjoy so you'll stick with it. At least once a week, work up a sweat and get your heart going for about an hour.

■ Regular checkups. If you're between 20 and 39, have your doctor examine your breasts every three years or so. She may opt to check more often depending on your history. After 40, you should have annual breast exams. If a lump is detected, don't panic. Most lumps are not cancerous. And remember, if cancer rears its ugly head, early detection is your best defense.

Simple way to slash your risk

Early detection of breast cancer still remains the best way to beat this ravaging disease. And when it comes to early detection, you hold the most important key. "Me?" you ask. "What about mammograms and all those other medical tests?"

Mammograms and yearly breast exams at your doctor's office are great ways to detect early cases of breast cancer. For the same reason, your monthly breast self-examination could be even more important for your breasts' health.

Chances are, you can detect changes in your breasts long before a doctor ever could, just because you are familiar with what is "normal" for you. Monthly breast self-examinations are a must for all women, regardless of age.

Here are answers to some common questions about examining your breasts.

■ **What am I looking for in these exams?** Quite simply, you are looking for any changes from what is "normal" for you. This could include lumps or knots in the breast tissue, any discharge from the nipple, or any change in the skin, such as dimpling or puckering. Call your doctor if you notice any changes.

■ **When is the best time to do these monthly exams?** If you're still having monthly menstrual cycles, the best time is one or two days after your period starts. That's when your breasts will be the least lumpy or tender from monthly changes. If you're past the age of menopause, just pick a day (the 1st, 15th, or 30th) each month that you can remember and stick with it. If you are taking hormones, talk with your doctor about when to do breast self-examinations.

■ **If you have naturally lumpy breasts, should you perform monthly breast exams anyway?** The answer is a hearty "yes." Even though lumpy breasts are a little more difficult to examine, and it's a little harder to notice new lumps or changes, you will be better at it than anyone else, just because you know your own lumps. Take a little extra time each month to get to know your "normal" lumps so you'll know when an "abnormal" lump shows up.

■ **If I am over age 50 and get yearly mammograms, can I stop performing monthly breast self-examinations?** Absolutely not! Mammograms are not foolproof. Nothing can replace your monthly self-examinations. You might find something six months before your next mammogram – that's too long to wait for a mammogram to pick it up. No matter how old you are or how often you get mammograms, you need to perform monthly breast self-examinations.

How to do a breast self-exam

1. Stand in front of a mirror that is large enough for you to see your breasts clearly. Check each breast for anything unusual. Check the skin for puckering, dimpling, or scaliness. Look for a discharge from the nipples.

Do steps 2 and 3 to check for any change in the shape or contour of your breasts. As you do these steps, you should feel your chest muscles tighten.

2. Watching closely in the mirror, clasp your hands behind your head and press your hands forward.

3. Next, press your hands firmly on your hips and bend slightly toward the mirror as you pull your shoulders and elbows forward.

4. Gently squeeze each nipple and look for a discharge.

5. Raise one arm. Use the pads of the fingers of your other hand to check the breast and the surrounding area firmly, carefully, and thoroughly. Some women like to use lotion or powder to help their fingers glide easily over the skin. Feel for any unusual lump or mass under the skin. Feel the tissue by pressing your fingers in small, overlapping areas about the size of a dime. To be sure you cover your whole breast, take your time and follow a definite pattern: lines, circles, or wedges.

Some research suggests that many women do breast self-examination more thoroughly when they use a pattern of up-and-down lines or strips. Other women, however, feel more comfortable with another pattern.

The important thing is to cover the whole breast and to pay special attention to the area between the breast and underarm, including the underarm itself. Check the area above the breast, up to the collarbone, and all the way over to your shoulder.

■ Lines: Start in the underarm area and move your fingers downward little by little until they are below the breast. Then move your fingers slightly toward the middle and slowly move back up. Go up and down until you cover the whole area.

■ Circles: Beginning at the outer edge of your breast, move your fingers slowly around the whole breast in a circle. Move around the breast in smaller and smaller circles, gradually working toward the nipple. Don't forget to check the underarm and upper chest areas too.

■ Wedges: Starting at the outer edge of the breast, move your fingers toward the nipple and back to the edge. Check your whole breast, covering one small wedge-shaped section at a time. Be sure to check your underarm area, as well as your upper chest.

6. It's important to repeat step 5 while you are lying down. Lie flat on your back, with one arm over your head and a pillow or folded towel under the opposite shoulder. This position flattens the breast and makes it easier for you to examine. Make sure you check each breast and the area around it very carefully using one of the patterns described previously.

7. Some women repeat step 5 in the shower. Your fingers will glide easily over soapy skin so you can concentrate on feeling for changes underneath.

If you notice a lump, a discharge, or any other change during the month, whether or not it is during breast self-examination, contact your doctor.

Surprising news about breast cancer

◆ A study at Georgetown University Medical Center found that women who are less educated about breast cancer are more likely to be frightened by breast cancer risk counseling and actually have mammograms less often.

◆ Certain professions may increase your risk of developing breast cancer. In a 20-year study of more than a million women in Sweden, pharmacists, telephone operators, hairdressers, doctors, religious workers, social workers, bank tellers, systems analysts, and computer programmers all had higher percentages of breast cancer than other professions. Although the exact cause is not known, some experts think the cancer may be related to radiation, electromagnetic fields, or lack of exercise. If you are in a high-risk job, be sure to monitor your breast health carefully.

◆ Women at risk of breast cancer are usually more anxious about their breast health and more likely to conduct frequent self-exams. While most experts recommend a monthly self-exam, research shows that many women check their breasts weekly, even daily. This is fine as long as you perform a thorough exam. Frequent, but quick, self-exams are more likely to miss critical changes in breast tissue. So take your time and do it right.

◆ Find a doctor who will take your symptoms – lumps, pain, nipple discharge, and skin changes – seriously. Studies show that more than 4 percent of women who complain about these symptoms are eventually diagnosed with breast cancer. Even if initial tests come back negative, ongoing symptoms should raise warning flags.

◆ If you are diagnosed with breast cancer and have a choice, go to a hospital that does a lot of breast cancer surgery. Studies show that your odds of survival are much higher.

Burns

6 ways to prevent burns

The next time you're racing around your kitchen trying to get dinner ready, remember this. Cooking fires are the leading cause of fires in the home. And burns are the second leading cause of accidental death.

If you are an older person, especially one with poor vision or arthritis, you need to take extra precautions. You can prevent most burns by thinking ahead and following these tips.

- Don't wear loose clothing when using the stove. Bathrobes with long, floppy sleeves are especially dangerous.

- Wear clothing you can remove quickly if it catches fire. Dresses and tops that open down the front and have Velcro fasteners rather than buttons are easier to get out of safely.

- If your clothing catches fire, stop, sit down, and calmly pat out the fire. Frantic movements can fan the flames and make your injuries worse.

- Cook on an electric rather than a gas stove to avoid the danger of flames. Use plug-in appliances, like tea kettles and small ovens, instead of the stove when possible.

- Be careful of food cooked in a microwave oven. It can be cool on the surface but scalding hot in the middle. Containers, too, can feel comfortable to the touch, while the food inside may be burning hot.

- To prevent scalding from hot water, have a plumber or electrician lower the temperature setting on your water heater. Most are set at 140 degrees. Water that hot can cause a third degree burn – the worst kind – in only 5 seconds. At 120 degrees, it takes 3 minutes of contact to do the same.

Adults over age 60 get burned more often than younger adults, and their burns tend to be larger as well. With care, you can avoid most of them. But if you do burn yourself, get help immediately. If you're alone, call 911.

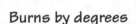

Burns by degrees

First-degree burns involve only the top layers of skin and usually leave no scars. The skin appears red and turns white when you touch it.

Second-degree burns look white or white with some redness, and they feel wet or waxy dry. Flames are often the cause of second-degree burns, and they usually do scar. You might not be able to tell the difference between a deep second-degree burn and a third-degree burn. If you're not sure, go ahead and see your doctor. He'll treat the burn in the office and show you how to care for it at home.

Third-degree burns usually look white or charred. You will only be able to feel deep pressure in a third-degree burn. The nerves are destroyed so you can't feel pain. You must see your doctor for these burns.

Sure-fire remedies

The pan slips as you are taking your favorite chocolate chip cookies out of the oven. Without thinking, you grab it with your bare hand. Ouch!

Before you do anything else, run cold water over the burn. Cold water helps relieve the pain. It's also the best way to stop the burning, which prevents damage to the skin and deeper layers of tissue.

Continue holding the burn under the running water – or press a cold, wet cloth to the area – until the pain goes away. It may take from 10 to 45 minutes. If you get a burn and water isn't available, use any cold liquid that's clean enough to drink.

Once you've cooled your injury, you need to decide if you should see a doctor. Here are some guidelines to help you. They come from Dr. Scott Dinehart, dermatologist and associate professor in the Department of Dermatology at the University of Arkansas.

Pay attention to how you are feeling. Serious burns can affect your overall health, not just where you were injured. "If you get a burn," says Dinehart, "and as a result are feeling sick – running a fever or just feeling bad in general – that would be a good sign to see a physician."

Beware of blisters. If you get a single blister, you probably don't need to worry. But if you get a lot of water-filled bubbles at the site of the burn, Dinehart suggests a visit to your doctor.

Size up the injury. A burn the size of your palm or bigger may be serious. Call your doctor.

Watch out for danger signals. "If you see signs of infection, like extreme warmth around the area, fever, or pus, you want to check with your physician," says Dinehart.

If you require medical care, your doctor may prescribe medication. For less serious burns, Dinehart says NSAIDs (nonsteroidal anti-inflammatory drugs), like aspirin or ibuprofen, can help relieve symptoms and decrease inflammation.

To care for your burn, wash it gently with a mild soap and warm water and coat it with an antibiotic cream. Never put butter or any other nonsterile grease on your burn. Cover the burned area lightly with gauze. Wash the burn and change the dressing once or twice a day.

Don't pop a blister. It's nature's way of protecting the burned tissue. If a blister does break, cover the area with a thin layer of antibiotic ointment.

Cancer

Choose to be cancer free

With the right tools, your body might be able to protect itself from cancer. Experts believe now, more than ever, you have the power to live a cancer-free life. When you choose to eat a balanced diet, exercise, and avoid smoking and drinking, you'll be choosing a lifestyle for cancer prevention.

Start by eating mostly plant-based foods. According to the American Cancer Society, balancing your diet this way could cut your cancer risk by one-third. Limit meats, fatty and sugary foods, and other empty calorie snacks. Punch up your intake of fruits, vegetables, legumes, and whole-grain breads and cereal. The nutrients, antioxidants, and fiber in these foods can help your body work smoothly, down to the last cell. And that's where it matters, because cancer starts when just one cell stops working properly.

Remember, the best cancer fighters aren't contained in hard-to-swallow pills but in colorful, flavorful foods. Here are the best food sources for cancer-proofing your body.

Antioxidants. Fruits, vegetables, and other plant-based foods are powerful weapons in the war against cancer. They're loaded with antioxidants, which are natural chemicals that reinforce your own anti-cancer defenses by fighting free radicals. Since free radicals can invade your cells and encourage cancer, all antioxidants are essential ammunition.

Many fruits and vegetables contain the big three – vitamin C, vitamin E, and beta carotene. Then again, some come armed to the teeth with even more antioxidants, like flavonoids. These compounds give color, flavor, and taste to plants. Your best bet is to load your plate with these superheroes.

■ Cruciferous vegetables. Also known as brassicas, this group includes broccoli, cauliflower, cabbage, kale, bok choy, kohlrabi, rutabaga, turnips, and brussels sprouts. These vegetables are famous for containing phytochemicals with long names like isothiocyanates, indoles, and glucosinolates. These natural substances appear to safeguard your DNA from cancer-causing mutations. They might even stop the growth of tumors. You'll get the most cancer protection if you eat these veggies raw or only lightly cooked.

■ Onions and garlic. These fragrant bulb vegetables, called alliums, also include scallions and chives. Mince or crush them to release their full anti-cancer powers, and don't overcook them. Follow these tips and you'll benefit from their flavonoids and sulfur compounds, which get free radicals before they get you.

■ Citrus fruits. Oranges, lemons, limes, grapefruits – these flavorful fruits are a two-for-one deal against cancer. Their pulp and juice are loaded with vitamin C. This amazing antioxidant might prevent more than eight different kinds of cancer in one fell swoop: cancers of the bladder, breast, cervix, colon and rectum, esophagus, lung, pancreas, and stomach. Plus, citrus fruits have antioxidants called monoterpenes in their peels. Shave off some of the fruit's outer skin, or zest, and add it to drinks or dishes for extra benefits.

■ Berries. According to the USDA-ARS Human Nutrition Research Center on Aging, these little morsels pack one of the biggest antioxidant punches. Natural chemicals like anthocyanin and ellagic acid deliver blows to cancer-causing pollutants. So eat strawberries, blueberries, cranberries, and other fruits that are so "berry" good for you.

■ Green leafies. Most vegetables with big floppy leaves and a dark green color, like romaine lettuce, collards, beet leaves, and spinach, contain carotenoids. These high-powered antioxidants take out toxins and free radicals before they can harm your cells. Carotenoids are especially powerful against lung cancer. So passive smokers take note – green leafies, as well as carrots and sweet potatoes, might be the protection you need from those pollutants you inhale.

■ Tomatoes. Lycopene is an antioxidant that sets tomatoes and other red fruits apart. This carotenoid appears to protect against cancers of the colon, stomach, lung, esophagus, prostate, and throat. Get as much lycopene as possible by sautéing tomatoes in olive oil, or by eating tomato-rich pasta sauces and pizza. Snacking on red grapefruit, guava, and watermelon will also lift your lycopene levels.

■ Herbs and spices. Use these cancer-fighters instead of salt to spice up your meals. Basil, rosemary, turmeric, ginger, and parsley all contain flavonoids and other compounds that send your antioxidant levels through the roof. Fresh herbs are generally more potent cancer fighters than dried.

This list is not complete. Dozens of foods contain antioxidants that ward off cancer. Don't forget green tea's polyphenols. Or olive oil's vitamin E. And there's the alpha and beta carotene in carrots. Load up your grocery cart with antioxidant power and start challenging the threat of cancer.

Selenium. This trace mineral is also an antioxidant, in that it protects your cells and tissues from oxidation. For nearly 30 years, scientists have believed low selenium levels lead to a greater risk of cancer. Selenium is different from other antioxidants, however, because a normal diet of mostly unprocessed foods easily provides the suggested 55 micrograms a day.

Now, Dr. Mark A. Nelson, a professor and researcher at the Arizona Cancer Center, says, "The Nutritional Prevention of Cancer (NPC) Trial tripled the intake and suggests that higher levels of selenium may be necessary for cancer prevention." Until nutritionists conduct more research, no one can recommend the best, safest amount you should get. Many health experts warn that selenium is a toxic mineral, which means too much of it, especially from supplements, is unsafe.

For now, Nelson's advice: "Eat a well-balanced diet." Foods especially high in selenium include mushrooms, seafood, chicken, broccoli, cabbage, and wheat.

"Grilling meats, poultry or — to a lesser degree — seafood has been linked to the risk of breast, stomach, and colorectal cancer," warns Melanie Polk of the American Institute for Cancer Research. But if you can't bear to give up that flame-broiled steak or burger, reduce your risk by marinating meats for at least 40 minutes.

Mix together three ingredients, an acidic liquid (like orange juice, wine, or vinegar), a flavoring (like turmeric or garlic), and something to hold everything together (like honey or olive oil). This helps prevent the cancer-causing compounds formed during grilling.

Folate. Folate is an essential ingredient in making DNA. Without enough of this incredible B vitamin, you could end up with broken chromosomes, which is a risk factor for cancer.

It's no wonder a folate deficiency could increase your risk for cancers of the cervix, lung, esophagus, brain, pancreas, breast – and especially the colon and rectum.

Munch on a salad made with fresh, leafy green vegetables to get more folate. Fortified cereals, beets, squash, and melon all provide a healthy amount, too. Eat these foods raw or lightly cooked since heat destroys the folate. Even microwaving will foil your folate intake.

Fiber. Dr. Denis Burkitt, author of *Eat Right – To Stay Healthy and Enjoy Life More*, first stated over 20 years ago that fiber might prevent colorectal cancer. "When diets are rich in dietary fiber," Burkitt said, "the stools passed are usually large. If carcinogens (substances that can cause cancer) are diluted in a large volume of stool and also if they are discarded out of the bowel fairly quickly (as happens with fiber-rich diets) rather than hanging around, they will be less dangerous."

Choose foods rich in insoluble fiber, the kind that won't dissolve in water. Good sources include brown rice, fruits, beans, vegetables, wheat bran, and whole grains. These are also rich in nutrients and phytochemicals, making them unbeatable anti-cancer weapons.

Omega-3. Your body needs two fatty acids that it can't make on its own — linolenic or omega-3 and linoleic or omega-6. They're called essential nutrients and you must get them from foods. But you must get them in correct amounts. When one type of fatty acid drastically outnumbers the other, things can go haywire.

Most people get more than enough omega-6 fatty acids from a typical diet loaded with vegetable oils, and not enough omega-3s. These fatty acids are found mainly in cold-water fish. Some experts believe this imbalance is linked to cancerous tumors. Too many omega-6 fatty acids may promote tumor growth, while getting more omega-3 fatty acids could prevent, and even shrink, tumors.

Win the battle between the omega-3s and the omega-6s. Every week eat at least two servings of salmon, tuna, mackerel, herring, or other omega-3-packed fish. Include flaxseeds, walnuts, and green leafy vegetables in your diet to boost your good fat intake even more. And just as important — cut back on eggs, milk, processed grains, and anything that contains corn or soybean oils. That includes almost all fried foods, fast foods, and margarine. These foods are all high in omega-6s.

Cut back on red meats, too. They're high in fats, including omega-6s and saturated fats. According to the American Cancer Society, a high-fat diet increases your risk of colon, rectal, prostate, and endometrial (uterine) cancers.

You can cut your risk even more by exercising. Healthy eating combined with exercise will help control your weight. If you are 20 to 30 percent over the ideal weight for your age, sex, and height, you are considered obese and that carries its own risks. Obese women are more likely to get cancer of the breast, uterus, ovary, and gallbladder. For obese men, it's colon and prostate cancer.

In addition to choosing healthier foods and exercising, if you cut out smoking and drinking, you could prevent up to 70 percent of all cancers. No wonder health experts say cancer prevention is in your hands.

Enjoy apricots for a long life

Believe it or not, some people claim apricots are the secret to living to age 120. They get this idea from the Hunzas, a tribe living in the Himalayan Mountains of Asia. Common health problems, like cancer, heart disease, high blood pressure, and high cholesterol, don't exist in Hunza. And researchers are wondering if apricots, a main part of their diet, are partly responsible. The Hunzas eat fresh apricots in season and dry the rest to eat during their long, cold winter.

The apricot is a fantastic fruit – loaded with beta carotene, iron, fiber, vitamin C, B vitamins, lycopene, magnesium, and copper. If you dry an apricot, its nutrients get more concentrated, making dried apricots a great snack.

Although eating apricots can't guarantee you'll live a long life, recent research suggests the little fruit may help you live a better life. The B vitamins in dried apricots may protect you from Alzheimer's and age-related mental problems, like memory loss.

It just goes to show how food is more powerful than pills when it comes to promoting a long, healthy life.

Canker sores

Soothe an irritated mouth naturally

Are painful canker sores making you feeling cantankerous? These unpleasant sores usually erupt inside the lip or cheek, or on the tongue, making life miserable. Fortunately, they are not contagious and usually heal within several weeks.

In the meantime, try not to fan the flames. Cool down hot foods before eating them. Avoid anything acidic, salty, spicy, or sugary, like tomatoes and tomato sauce, pickled foods, hot peppers, and citrus fruits. Watch out for foods with sharp edges, like potato chips, that can further irritate your sores. Use a straw to avoid contact if you drink carbonated beverages.

Beat the heat with milk. During an outbreak, drinking cold milk with your food can soothe the pain of canker sores. Just swish a mouthful around and swallow from time to time during your meal. You may be able to prevent canker sores by eating from four tablespoons to two cups of plain live-culture yogurt a day. Be sure to buy the kind that contains *lactobacillus acidophilus*, a bacterium that helps keep your immune system healthy.

Treat with tea and vitamin E. A quick fix for the pain of a canker sore is as easy as a cup of tea – without the cup. Simply hold a wet tea bag in your mouth over the sore. Adjust the bag from time to time for comfort, but keep it over the sore for at least 10 minutes. Tannin, a natural substance found in black tea, is an astringent that will help dry up and heal the sore. Dandelion tea may also heal the sores and prevent their return.

For early treatment, punch a hole in a vitamin E capsule and squeeze the gel directly on the sores as soon as they appear. This can be repeated from time to time until they are healed.

Swish away pain. A good gargle can work wonders, too. Some studies suggest that certain bacteria in your mouth make it easier for sores to form. A solution of three parts water to one part hydrogen peroxide can help keep your mouth clean and make it harder for bacteria to grow. You might want to try a few of these herbal mouthwashes as well.

- Goldenseal, known for its ability to kill certain bacteria, can soothe and heal canker sores. Make a mouth rinse by mixing 6 grams (two teaspoons) of goldenseal in a cup of boiling water. After it cools, rinse your mouth several times a day.

- Myrrh is another antibacterial that usually comes in an alcohol solution. You can use it directly on the sores or rinse your mouth with it. To make a mouthwash, mix five to 10 drops of the myrrh solution in a glass of water.

- Sage makes a good mouthwash for canker sores because it has both antiseptic and anti-inflammatory qualities. Add two teaspoons of finely cut sage to a cup of boiling water, mix, and cool before using.

- Geranium and lavender oils, one drop of each mixed with a half cup of water, make an aromatic mouthwash that can be used four times a day.

- Deglycyrrhizinated liquorice mouthwash was tested in India on 20 people with canker sores. Fifteen subjects found a 50 to 75 percent improvement within one day, and their sores were completely healed within three days. The glycyrrhizine is removed from this form of licorice. That ingredient can cause serious side effects, especially for people with high blood pressure and heart problems. Unfortunately, most so-called licorice candy made in the United States is actually flavored with anise.

4 common causes of canker sores

Allergies crank 'em up. It's a fact, certain foods and drinks often trigger canker sores in some people. Among the most common are chocolate, seeds, nuts, gelatin, alcohol, and anything spicy or acidic. In one study of 21 people with canker sores, 20 had food allergies. After being told what to avoid, 18 subjects reported an improvement in their condition. To prevent canker sores, try to figure out if you're allergic to certain foods. You may see an improvement in your own condition as well.

Sensitive to cinnamon? This spice is one of the worst culprits when it comes to causing canker sores. You may already avoid red-hot candies, cinnamon-flavored chewing gum, and cinnamon buns. But it also hides in foods like cookies, cereals, chili, and flavored teas and coffees. What's more, it's sometimes added to mouthwashes, toothpastes, and breath fresheners to make them taste better. To avoid an unpleasant surprise, be sure to check foods label for this spicy ingredient.

Canker sores usually appear in places that come in direct contact with cinnamon. People who frequently suck on hard candies tend to get them on one side of the tongue or cheek. Cinnamon tea drinkers, on the other hand, are more likely to get them through out the mouth.

"B" alert and iron out deficiencies. What if you've given up everything that has any flavor and still suffer from painful sores? Maybe you're not getting enough iron and B vitamins, especially folic acid and B12. A lack of these seems to be a main cause of recurrent canker sores.

Eating lots of beef liver is one way to get enough of all three, but there are other, perhaps more tempting, alternatives. A good source of iron and folic acid is green leafy vegetables. To get both vitamin B12 and folic acid, try chicken livers. Another good source of B12 is fish, especially sardines, crab, herring, and salmon. Other missing B vitamins may lead to canker sores, too. You may be low in B1 (thiamin), found in pork, beans, nuts, egg yolks, wheat germ, and oatmeal; B2 (riboflavin), found in fish, poultry, milk, and green vegetables; or B6 (pyridoxine) found in avocados, bananas, chicken, turkey, and sunflower seeds.

Zero in on zinc. Your canker sores could be caused by a zinc deficiency. One study involved a 15-year-old boy who suffered with canker sores for six years. He was treated with a variety of medications, but the sores kept coming back. When doctors found he was deficient in zinc, they gave him 50 milligrams (mg) of zinc sulfate by mouth three times a day. After three months, the canker sores disappeared and did not come back for a year.

Before taking high doses of zinc supplements, have your blood tested to see if you have a zinc deficiency. The recommended dietary allowance for a healthy adult male over age 50 is 11 milligrams (mg). For women, it's 8 mg. Most experts suggest that 50 mg a day is the most you should take even to restore a zinc deficiency.

The best food sources of zinc are beef, oysters and other seafood, poultry, beans, and whole grains.

Do cankers lead to cancer?

If you're a canker sore sufferer who loves beer and hot dogs, you may want to rethink your choice of refreshments.

Beer and hot dogs contain nitrites, and research has shown that nitrites can turn into nitrosamines and cause cancer. Studies also show that people who get canker sores and eat a lot of nitrites are seven times more likely than average to get cancer of the esophagus.

But the good news is black tea and vitamin C seem to prevent nitrites from breaking down into cancer-causing nitrosamines. So you may want to drink iced tea or lemonade with those hot dogs instead of beer.

Nitrites are also found in smoked fish and processed meats, like ham, bacon, sausage, and luncheon meats. You can also balance your nitrites with extra vitamin C by having a glass of orange juice with your breakfast bacon or sausage. Put lettuce and tomato on a ham sandwich. Keep a shaker of vitamin C sprinkles handy and add them freely at the table.

Vegetables contain nitrites, too. But they have other substances that prevent the breakdown of nitrites into nitrosamines. In fact, eating fresh vegetables actually seems to lower your risk of getting cancer.

Chances are, canker sores won't increase your risk of cancer. But it's still a good idea to eat more fresh vegetables and fewer processed meats.

Carpal tunnel syndrome

Protect your wrists from strain and pain

Variety is the spice of life. Never is that saying more true than for someone suffering from carpal tunnel syndrome. If your work or hobby involves repeating a certain motion with your hands, tendons in your wrist can swell, pinching a nerve and causing pain. Changing the way you do things will not only spice up your life, it might prevent wrist pain.

There are many names for it – tendonitis, repetitive motion injury, cumulative trauma disorder. Whether you type, sew, drive a bus, cut hair, operate power tools, or play a musical instrument, you are at risk.

You might have carpal tunnel syndrome if your fingers, hands, or wrists become weak; you have numbness, tingling, or burning in your hands or fingers; or you have pain that travels up your arm, especially at night.

Some people resort to surgery to ease the pressure on the nerve, but, unfortunately, surgery has side effects and very often the symptoms reappear. Your best plan is to prevent carpal tunnel syndrome in the first place.

Try a wrist workout. Experts from the American Academy of Orthopaedic Surgeons say carpal tunnel syndrome can be prevented by regularly stretching and exercising your wrists. They advise you to get in the habit of doing exercises like these several times a day.

■ Take a break every hour and vigorously shake your hands for about 15 seconds. This relieves cramped muscles and gets your blood flowing.

■ Hold your arms straight out in front of you, palms down. Bend your wrists up until your palms are facing front and you feel a nice, easy stretch in your forearms. Repeat this several times.

■ Make your hand into a tight fist. Bend your wrist down to stretch your forearm. Straighten your wrist and open up your hand, fanning your fingers out as far apart as possible. Hold and repeat several times.

■ Sit with your forearm resting on the arm of your chair. With your opposite hand, grab your fingers and pull them so your wrist is gently stretched back. Hold this position for about 15 seconds. Then let your wrist relax so your fingers are pointing toward the ground. Gently push on the back of your hand so your wrist and forearm are stretched down. Hold for 15 seconds. Repeat several times with each hand.

Watch how you sit. The majority of people suffering from carpal tunnel syndrome spend many hours at a computer. Although there are hundreds of products designed for computer users to ease wrist strain, such as ergonomic keyboards and mice, some experts think this near-epidemic of wrist injury is the result of how you sit, not the position of your hands.

No matter what you are doing, when you sit, your posture naturally follows how your head and upper arms are positioned. Keeping them in line with your spine and hips forces your back, shoulders, abdomen, forearms, and hands to stay in a stress-free position.

When you're sitting, whether it's in front of a computer or a sewing machine, don't let your head or upper arms reach forward. Keep your chest directly over your pelvis, with your diaphragm and stomach muscles tightened and lifted.

When you're using a keyboard, your weight should not be on your wrists. This increases the pressure on the nerves in your wrists. That's why wrist supports may not relieve carpal tunnel syndrome. If your body is positioned properly, you won't need to support your wrists at all. They will simply glide over the keys with an easy, relaxed arm motion.

Be kind to your wrists. Remember, you don't have to sit in front of a computer to suffer from carpal tunnel syndrome. It can come from any activity that involves doing the same thing over and over again with your hands. Even something as relaxing as gardening or woodworking can cause this physical stress. To avoid turning a favorite pastime into a painful chore, follow these wrist-saving tips:

■ Change tasks every 30 minutes.

■ Take a break between tasks. Run through a few of the hand exercises mentioned previously.

■ Don't lean your weight on your hands. Work in a position where your body weight is supported by stronger joints.

■ Choose carefully. Buy tools that have padded handles or are ergonomically designed.

■ Put shock absorbers on power tools.

■ Keep your grip on objects as loose and relaxed as possible.

■ Change positions frequently.

■ Use electrical devices that will save your hands, like power staplers, tillers, etc.

■ Use as little force as possible to get the job done. Typing with a light touch can correct carpal tunnel syndrome.

Cataracts

Nutritional ABCs can save your sight

According to the American Academy of Ophthalmology, cataracts strike nearly everyone by age 75. But just by eating the right things, and avoiding the harmful ones, you can protect yourself from cataracts and other vision problems.

Ante up with vitamin A. The first of three protective antioxidant vitamins gets top billing when it comes to helping your eyes. Vitamin A guards against free radical damage that can lead to night blindness, cataracts, and macular degeneration. High doses of vitamin A have even been used by doctors to successfully treat a rare genetic eye disorder called Sorsby's fundus dystrophy, which can cause blindness.

Meats and dairy products contain vitamin A, but your body converts plant substances called carotenoids, such as beta carotene, lutein, and zeaxanthin, into vitamin A, too.

Choose bright yellow or orange fruits and vegetables, like apricots, mangoes, carrots, and sweet potatoes, for beta carotene. Green, leafy vegetables, like spinach and collard greens, will give you plenty of lutein and zeaxanthin.

Be smart about B vitamins. It's not just antioxidant vitamins that protect your eyes. Researchers conducting the Blue Mountain Eye Study discovered that people deficient in niacin, thiamin, and riboflavin, very important members of the B-vitamin family, were more likely to get nuclear cataracts. This kind of cataract affects the central part of your lens. Fortunately, eating a bowl of fortified breakfast cereal will give you all three of these important nutrients. Other excellent sources include tuna, whole-wheat bread, baked potatoes, and mushrooms.

See better with C. Vitamin C, another antioxidant, also plays a role in protecting your eyes from free radicals. Oranges, lemons, tangerines, strawberries, cantaloupe, broccoli, brussels sprouts, and sweet red peppers are great sources of vitamin C.

Eat enough E. Eating vitamin E-rich foods every day can cut your risk of getting cataracts in half. Just like vitamin A, vitamin E counteracts the harmful free radicals produced by exposure to light and oxygen. You can find vitamin E in wheat germ, sunflower seeds, nuts, whole grains, and brown rice.

Pay attention to protein. Chances are, you get enough protein from the meat, fish, and dairy products in your diet. But a protein deficiency could put you at greater risk for nuclear cataracts. If you're a vegetarian, this is a real concern. Make sure you mix your vegetable proteins, which are "incomplete" by themselves, to maximize your protection. Here's a good example – eat beans with rice and enjoy peanut butter with whole-grain bread.

Spare the salt. A high-salt diet could mean high risk for your eyes. In fact, in one study, those whose diet included about 3,000 milligrams (mg) of salt a day were twice as likely to develop cataracts as those getting only about 1,000 mg a day. Try using herbs instead of salt to flavor your food. Garlic and onions improve almost any meal, and turmeric might even improve your eyesight. This spice, often used in Indian curry dishes, contains curcumin, an antioxidant that helped fight off cataracts in animal studies. It's also a good idea to avoid fast foods and read the labels before buying processed foods, which are usually high in sodium.

Ditch the fat. Choose lean meats and low-fat dairy products and avoid foods high in saturated fats, like egg yolks, whole milk, cheese, lard, butter, coconut oil, palm oil, and hydrogenated vegetable oils.

Protecting your vision doesn't have to be complicated. As you plan your meals from day to day, just remember – how you eat affects how you see.

Thwart sight-stealers with sweet melons

Worried about your eyesight? Reach for a cantaloupe.

Cantaloupes are full of beta carotene, a carotenoid your body converts into vitamin A. This natural chemical not only gives the melon its brilliant orange color, but it also acts as an antioxidant in your body, protecting your eyes from serious problems like cataracts and macular degeneration

These two serious eye problems most often strike seniors. Cataracts blind over 1 million people worldwide every year, and age-related macular degeneration (AMD) is the leading cause of blindness in people over age 65. But you can guard against both diseases by eating the right foods.

Australian researchers conducting the Blue Mountain Eye Study found that people who took in at least 3,000 retinol equivalents (RE) of vitamin A a day cut their risk of developing nuclear cataracts, the kind that affects the central area of your lens, in half.

Although this amount of vitamin A is more than the recommended dietary allowance (RDA), it's still a safe level as long as you're getting the vitamin from whole foods, not supplements. Eat one small cantaloupe a day, and you're halfway to this sight-saving goal.

Antioxidants like beta carotene may safeguard your retina from free radical damage, and they also help keep the blood vessels surrounding your eye working properly, all factors that protect against AMD.

According to studies out of five major ophthalmology centers, the more carotenoids like beta carotene you eat, the lower your risk of developing this disease.

Vitamin C, plentiful in cantaloupe, is another antioxidant superpower. Eat one small cantaloupe, containing over 180 milligrams of vitamin C, every day, and you could cut your risk of developing macular degeneration by one-third.

More natural ways to discourage cataracts

While age is the number one cause of cataracts, there are lifestyle choices you can make to decrease your risk.

Protect your eyes from the sun. Experts agree – if you spend too much time in the sun without protecting your eyes, you're at higher risk of developing eye diseases, like cataracts.

When buying sunglasses, make sure you select a pair that block at least 99 percent of ultraviolet (UV) light. If the label says "UV absorption up to 400 nm," that means the same thing. Don't worry about protection from infrared light. The latest research hasn't shown any connection between eye problems and the relatively low levels found in sunlight.

Amber, polarized, and mirrored lenses can make a difference in how well you see during different outdoor activities, but they don't have anything to do with protecting you from UV radiation. Neither does the color of the lenses nor how dark they are. Large, wrap-around styles are a good idea. They protect from all angles. Ordinary frames allow light to shine around the sides, over the tops, and into your eyes.

And remember – expensive doesn't necessarily mean better. You don't have to pay big bucks for good sunglasses. That $100 pair may have more style, but the $10 pair could be just as good, or better, for your eyes. UV protection is what matters most, not the price. To judge the quality of sunglasses, it helps to look at something with a rectangular pattern, like floor tile. Hold the glasses several inches from your face, cover one eye, and move the glasses from side to side and up and down. The lines should stay straight. Choose another pair if the lines look wavy, especially in the center.

If you take medication that makes your skin more sensitive to the sun, your eyes will be more sensitive, too. These photosensitizing drugs include tetracycline, doxycycline, and allopurinol. Talk to your ophthalmologist if you have any questions.

Stay away from cigarettes. Cigarette smoke can do more than cloud up a room. It can dim your eyesight as well. While experts may not be able to explain how it happens, they do know smokers are two to three times more likely to get cataracts than nonsmokers. Still, it's never too late to turn things around. By simply cutting out cigarettes, you'll be cutting your risk of cataracts, too.

Be aware of the aspirin controversy. Aspirin therapy for cataracts is still a controversial subject. While some studies indicate that taking aspirin might help prevent cataracts, more recent research shows long-term use of aspirin can actually increase your risk. Experts found that people who took one or more aspirin tablets a week for a period of 10 years were twice as likely to have cataracts as those who didn't take aspirin very often. This seemed to be truest for people under age 65.

In another large study, researchers found no evidence that taking low doses of aspirin every other day helped prevent cataracts. There is a possibility, however, that a treatment like this could decrease the number of cataract surgeries, a $2.5 billion annual expense in the United States. If aspirin therapy was able to postpone the need for surgery by several years, it could save millions of dollars in hospital bills. A word of caution – if you are taking aspirin for your heart or other health reasons, don't stop without your doctor's approval.

Ask your doctor about estrogen. Post-menopausal women are at high risk of developing cataracts. Animal studies at the Indiana University School of Medicine show hormone replacement therapy might help prevent cataracts in older women.

Say no to alcohol. Scientists have found where there is regular alcohol use, there is also a slightly higher rate of cataracts. And having a daily drink is a greater risk than drinking just once a month. While researchers continue to study this connection, you might want to cut back on alcohol.

Celiac disease

Change your menu for lasting relief

Celiac disease, also called celiac sprue, causes the hair-like villi of the small intestine to become inflamed and flattened. And since nutrients from food are absorbed through these tiny villi, the disease often leads to symptoms of malnutrition, even if you are eating healthy, well-balanced meals.

The culprit in celiac disease is gluten, and it's found in some of the most commonly eaten foods on earth – wheat, barley, rye, and oats. If you have celiac disease, you can't eat foods made from a variety of grains without damaging your small intestine.

And the stakes are high. Up to 15 percent of people with the disease develop gastrointestinal cancer or lymphoma. Yet, if you eat a gluten-free diet, you can usually recover from celiac disease completely, and your chances of getting cancer can return to normal.

Possible symptoms of celiac disease are weakness, anemia, bone pain, weight loss, stomach bloating, and diarrhea or bulky stools that float. All of these symptoms are a result of not getting nutrition from the foods you eat. In addition, celiac disease often leads to lactose intolerance, the inability to digest milk.

Other conditions that sometimes show up with celiac disease are dermatitis herpetiformis (burning, itching rashes that last for weeks or months), liver disease, juvenile diabetes, thyroid disease, lupus, rheumatoid arthritis, Sjogren's syndrome (very dry eyes and mouth), and ulcers of the mouth. But sometimes celiac disease has no symptoms at all, just harmful changes in your small intestine.

Celiac disease affects one in 300 people in Europe. It's especially prevalent in Italy and Ireland but rare in Africa, Japan, and China.

Doctors in the United States don't test for celiac disease very often, and many people with these symptoms are often told they have irritable bowel syndrome (IBS) or a nervous disorder. Children who have untreated celiac disease are often small for their age, but normal-size adults can develop it after severe stress, a viral infection, or pregnancy.

Researchers aren't sure if it's present from birth and then triggered, or if you can develop it later in life. Breast-fed children seem to have some protection against developing the disease at a young age. At this time, the only certain test for celiac disease is removal of a tiny piece of the small intestine to check for damage to the villi. If your doctor finds changes in your small intestine, and a totally gluten-free diet relieves your symptoms, chances are good you have the disease.

If you're diagnosed with celiac disease, you'll have to follow a strict, gluten-free diet for the rest of your life. Besides the obvious sources, like breads, gluten is found in all kinds of foods — sauces, gravies, candies, and many alcoholic drinks, like beer, gin, and whiskey. Ask questions in restaurants, and read labels in the grocery store. And if you're not sure, don't eat it.

People with celiac disease often have difficulty absorbing fat-soluble vitamins, like A, D, and K, and can be deficient in these and other nutrients. But once you cut all gluten foods out of your diet, your small intestine should begin to heal, and food can again be your ally instead of your enemy. If you have severe malnutrition, your doctor might prescribe supplements.

Here are some invaluable nutrition tips that can help you fight celiac disease.

Gluten-free flours. You'll have to completely avoid all breads and cereals containing wheat, rye, oats, barley, bran, graham, wheat germ, durum, kaska, bulgar, buckwheat, millet, triticale, amaranth, spelt, teff, quinoa, and kamut. Also off limits are malt and wheat starch, often used to thicken sauces. You can replace these with breads and cereals made from rice, corn, potato, and bean flour. Look for breads that are labeled "gluten-free" or make your own.

You'll have to be a food detective to avoid all sources of gluten in your diet. Some herbal teas and nondairy creamers contain gluten, as does tuna in vegetable broth and any hydrolyzed vegetable protein. Avoid creamed vegetables, raisins and dried dates that have been dusted with flour, most canned soups, and sauces.

Some types of cheeses, like blue, Roquefort, and Gorgonzola, are surprising sources of gluten. Even ketchup and soy sauce can contain gluten. For more help, find a dietitian and contact a support group for people with celiac disease.

Vitamin A. Symptoms of a vitamin A deficiency are night blindness, inflammation of the eyes, reduced ability to fight infection, weight loss, loss of appetite, reduced saliva, and improper tooth and bone formation. You can counteract these symptoms with whole milk (if you aren't lactose intolerant – a problem for many celiacs), yellow and dark green vegetables, oranges, and liver.

Vitamin D. If you don't get enough vitamin D, your body can't use calcium to make strong bones. Good sources are fatty fish, like salmon, herring, and sardines, and their oils. Eggs, butter, and liver are also good foods to eat to boost your levels of vitamin D naturally. Your body can also make vitamin D with the help of sunlight. But as you get older, the process doesn't work as well.

Vitamin K. This vitamin is important for proper blood clotting, and a lack of vitamin K can lead to anemia. Green leafy vegetables and liver are good sources.

Magnesium. If you have trouble absorbing nutrients, you could be deficient in the multi-talented mineral magnesium, especially if you've had diarrhea for a long time. Not having enough magnesium can cause muscle tremors, personality changes, nausea, vomiting, and even convulsions. Fill up on nuts, legumes, seafood, and green, leafy vegetables.

Calcium. Everyone needs calcium for healthy bones. If you are lactose intolerant, you can get calcium from yogurt, which is easier to digest than milk. Once you've been on a gluten-free diet for several months, you might be able to tolerate more milk products. Many celiacs find that lactose intolerance clears up as they get better.

Chronic fatigue syndrome

Uncover the mystery of chronic fatigue

Most people love a good mystery. Trying to figure out "whodunit" can be fun and relaxing. However, when the mystery is "why am I so tired all the time?" and not even your doctor has the answer, it is neither fun nor relaxing.

Everyone feels tired sometimes, but if you have persistent fatigue that lasts more than six months, and your doctor has ruled out other causes, you may have chronic fatigue immune dysfunction syndrome (CFIDS). Other symptoms of this mysterious disorder include mild fever, tender lymph nodes, sore throat, headaches, confusion, and muscle aches.

Diseases similar to chronic fatigue have battled doctors for over a century. Each generation has had different names and different possible causes for these disorders. They have been called neurasthenia, the yuppie flu, shirkers syndrome, and chronic EBV (Epstein Barr Virus). Possible causes include anemia, allergies, low blood sugar, yeast infections, viruses, and mental disorders.

CFIDS often begins after an illness, like a cold, bronchitis, or mononucleosis. Researchers still have not established a definite cause for CFIDS, but most now believe it is caused by a virus or by a malfunctioning immune system. Although CFIDS has no tried and true treatment or cure, researchers and people with the disorder have found some strategies that could help.

Heed amino acid advice. Some people with chronic fatigue syndrome have found that certain amino acids help ease their symptoms. Lysine is an amino acid that fights the herpes virus that causes cold sores and mouth ulcers. The same virus may play a role in CFIDS. L-carnitine might also help. It is a combination of lysine and methionine, another amino acid. Natural sources of lysine include eggs, fish, lima beans, red meat, potatoes, milk, cheese, and yeast. If you choose to take supplements, the recommended dosage is 1 to 2 grams daily.

Another amino acid, arginine, can undo lysine's hard work, so steer clear of it. Don't take any supplements that contain arginine, and try to limit your intake of arginine-rich foods, like chocolate, nuts, raisins, whole wheat, and brown rice.

Add pep with vitamins and minerals. With any chronic illness, your body's supply of essential vitamins and minerals can become drained. Magnesium levels seem to be particularly low in people with CFIDS, and supplementation with magnesium has improved symptoms in some people. A multi-vitamin/mineral supplement could help give you energy and keep your nutrient levels on an even keel.

Boost energy with herbs. Echinacea, a colorful flowering plant, was first used as medicine by Native Americans. Early settlers used this healing plant as treatment for everything from dizziness to rattlesnake bites.

Although echinacea's medicinal use declined after the discovery of antibiotics, modern research has found that echinacea can provide natural help for a sluggish immune system. And anything that gives your immune system a boost might boost your energy levels, too.

Ginseng, a root used as medicine for centuries in the Far East, may help pick you up and get you moving. Ginseng has reportedly been used to cure almost any illness you can imagine. Studies show that ginseng increases energy and helps your muscles work longer and more efficiently. Research also finds that ginseng helps your immune system produce more of the cells that attack infections.

One study tested the effects of echinacea and ginseng on people with chronic fatigue syndrome. Both herbs significantly increased the immune function of cells.

If you decide to try these herbal supplements, look for standardized ginseng supplements that contain 4 to 7 percent ginsenosides. The recommended dosage is 100 milligrams (mg) every day.

Echinacea is most commonly sold as a liquid extract. Experiment with the dosage to find what works best for you. For immune system boosting, many herbal experts recommend 10 to 25 drops of extract or one to two capsules a day. If you take echinacea for an extended period of time, it loses its effectiveness, so try taking it for three days on and three days off.

Find some fatty acids. Omega-3 and omega-6 fatty acids may be the end of the tired, aching muscles of CFIDS. These fatty acids may help reduce inflammation, pain, and flu-like symptoms. You can find these acids in evening primrose oil (omega-6) and fish oil (omega-3).

If these tips don't help your chronic fatigue, don't despair. CFIDS sometimes disappears just as mysteriously as it appeared. In the meantime, get some rest, eat well-balanced meals, and exercise regularly. And who knows? Research may soon uncover the solution to this medical mystery.

Colds and flu

Outsmart colds with healing foods

The old saying, "Feed a cold and starve a fever," may not be good advice. Eating certain foods can be great therapy for colds and flu, even if you have a fever.

In fact, research indicates that chicken soup – the world-famous cold remedy created with love by mothers everywhere – can help you feel better. The hot liquid moistens and clears your nasal passages and soothes your sore throat. And a recent study found that chicken soup can relieve symptoms of an upper respiratory tract infection by reducing inflammation.

Don't underestimate the emotional healing associated with chicken soup, either. When you're feeling miserable, a warm cup of soup can be very comforting.

And there's more. Some foods boost your immune system so you won't "come down" with the flu or "catch" a cold in the first place. So look through your cupboards. You're sure to find a variety of foods that can help speed your recovery and keep you healthy.

Garlic. Garlic won't do much for your breath, but it might help prevent cold and flu viruses from invading and damaging your tissues. This powerful herb may also bolster your immune system. And if you toss some garlic into your chicken soup, you'll be getting two natural infection fighters at the same time.

Water. To prevent dehydration, drink plenty of water, especially when you have a cold or the flu. Dr. Mary L. Hardy, director of the Integrative Medicine Medical Group at Cedars-Sinai Medical Center in Los Angeles, believes in the healing power of water. "The first defense system in the body consists of the mucous membranes lining the upper respiratory tract," she says. "And those work better when they're moist. Drink plenty of water and use steam treatments to provide internal and external hydration."

Vitamin C. Some people drink more orange juice the instant they feel the first sniffle or body ache – and it's probably a good idea. While vitamin C probably won't prevent colds, research shows it might shorten the length of time you suffer from cold symptoms. Guava, sweet red peppers, strawberries, grapefruit, oranges, lemons, limes, and cantaloupe are good sources of vitamin C.

Zinc. Getting enough of this mineral in your diet may help reduce your risk of infection caused by bacteria and viruses. Oysters are a great source of zinc, but if you're not a shellfish fan, you can also find it in chicken, beef, lamb, turkey, beans, barley, and wheat.

Beta carotene. If you don't get enough beta carotene in your diet, you might be more likely to get a cold or the flu. Beta carotene, which is converted into vitamin A by your body, helps you fight infections. To get beta carotene, eat brightly colored fruits and vegetables. Good sources include carrots, pumpkin, sweet potatoes, kale, spinach, apricots, cantaloupe, mangoes, and broccoli.

Ginger. Soothing a sore throat can be a snap with ginger. For centuries, this herb has battled several illnesses, including colds and the flu, and it may be particularly helpful in reducing mucus. To make a pot of comforting ginger tea, place three or four slices of the fresh root in a pint of hot water. Simmer for 10 to 30 minutes, and sip on the soothing concoction all day.

Echinacea. Native Americans have used this herb for hundreds of years to treat colds, coughs, sore throats, toothaches, and even snakebites. It seems to fight colds and flu by boosting your immune system. Most herbal experts agree it is helpful in treating the early stages of upper respiratory tract infections. However, there is no strong evidence it will help prevent them. You may have trouble deciding which echinacea product to use since even the clinical trials tested different doses, different species of echinacea, different types of preparations, and sometimes a combination of herbal products. The well-respected German commission E recommends taking 300 to 400 milligrams (mg) of dry echinacea extract three times a day.

Other herbal remedies used to fight colds include marshmallow root, slippery elm, mullein flower, licorice, elderberry, astragalus root, goldenseal root, wild cherry bark (tea or tincture), eucalyptus or camphor rub, honey and lemon, thyme, fenugreek, cayenne, and horseradish.

9 ways to survive the cold and flu season

Here are some simple tips for avoiding colds and flu – and for feeling better fast if you get sick anyway.

Sidestep stress. When you're under stress, your immune system doesn't work as well as it should. This makes your body more vulnerable to infections, including colds and flu. Try to get a handle on your problems by keeping your sense of humor and a healthy perspective. Eliminate the unimportant things in your life. Make time for the people and activities you really care about.

Wash your hands. You can catch a cold or the flu by touching something exposed to the virus, like someone's hand or a telephone, then touching your eyes, nose, or mouth. Once germs get into your respiratory system, they'll spread quickly. You can also get infected by inhaling particles in the air from a cough or sneeze.

To reduce your chances of getting sick, keep your hands away from your eyes, nose, and mouth, and wash them frequently. Use plain, liquid soap and rub your hands together vigorously for best results. Liquid soap is a better choice because bar soap can harbor germs. The popular antibacterial soaps don't provide protection against colds and flu because they only kill bacteria, not viruses.

Catch extra shut-eye. When your body is working to fight off a cold or the flu, it needs plenty of rest. Don't push yourself. Take a day off from your normal activities. It will help you get well, and it might protect your friends and co-workers from catching your germs and getting sick.

Bid germs farewell. Keep your house clean and germ free, and you'll protect yourself from colds and flu. Use a solution of bleach and water to clean kitchen counters, doorknobs, cabinet handles, staircase railings, telephones, and anything else you touch. Change pillowcases and hand towels often.

Calm your cough. You can make your own natural cough syrup by mixing the juice of one lemon with two tablespoons of glycerine and 12 teaspoons of honey. Take one teaspoon every half hour, stirring well before each use. For another soothing and tasty cough reliever, combine 8 ounces of warm pineapple juice and two teaspoons of honey.

Gargle. The best and most comforting gargle for your sore throat is warm, salty water. One-half teaspoon of salt stirred into a cup of warm water will make a soothing solution. Another good gargle is strong, brewed tea, which has an astringent, or drying, effect. You can gargle with it warm or cold.

Get steamed up. If a stuffy nose is making you miserable, try a little steam. The hot, moist air can temporarily clear clogged nasal passages and help you breathe easier. It also can prevent your sinuses from becoming dry and irritated, which could lead to swelling and infection. So jump in the shower, plug in a humidifier, or make your own private steam bath with boiling water in a bowl. Just cover your head with a towel, lean over the bowl, and breathe deeply. Add some chamomile flowers to the water to help clear clogged sinuses, calm your cough, and soothe your irritated throat. Or try adding pine oil, eucalyptus, or menthol for a little extra nasal-opening power.

If you can't slow down long enough to sit over a bowl, try this clever home remedy. Cut a strip from the bottom of an old T-shirt. Soak it in hot water or microwave the damp shirt until it's warm.

Tie it around your head, covering your nose. This gives you the same effect as sitting over a bowl of hot water, but it allows you the freedom to move around.

Keep your nose clean. A nasal wash or nasal irrigation is an excellent tool for fighting a cold or the flu. It washes bacteria and excess mucus from your sinuses and helps prevent a sinus infection. You'll need a large rubber syringe that you can buy at your local drugstore. Make a solution of one-half teaspoon of plain (not iodized) salt and a pinch of baking soda mixed with one cup of warm water.

Fill the syringe, then place it in one nostril and pinch the nostril closed around it. Squeeze the syringe to move the saline solution through your nose, then blow your nose gently. Most of the salty solution will come out through your mouth, so just rinse with plain water to remove it.

Continue until the drainage is clean, then repeat with the other nostril. To keep your nasal syringe from reinfecting you later, clean it well after every use. Store it on end in a clean glass so any remaining water can drain out. Don't share nasal syringes. Make sure every family member has his own.

Give hankies the heave-ho. With a cold or flu, you'll probably blow your nose a lot. Be sure to use disposable tissues instead of handkerchiefs. Then you won't reinfect yourself as you're getting well, and you're less likely to infect others. Dispose of dirty tissues carefully in a sealed bag.

Inject more power into your flu shot

Your next bout with influenza might be more than an inconvenience – it could be deadly. Although flu season affects everyone, it takes its toll on seniors. If you're over age 65, your odds of becoming seriously ill, or even dying, from the flu skyrocket. Getting a flu shot gives you the best protection, and doctors recommend it yearly for anyone over age 50. Try to get vaccinated between mid-October and mid-November, although you can do it anytime from September through March.

Experts estimate that if everyone got a flu shot as suggested, it would prevent 70 percent of hospitalizations and 80 percent of deaths related to the flu. By taking a few extra steps, you can protect yourself even further. Here's how to get the most out of your flu shot.

Grab some ginseng. A recent study found that taking 100 milligrams (mg) of this herbal supplement twice a day for four months enhanced the power of a flu shot. By giving your immune system a boost, ginseng reinforces your body's battle against the flu.

Relax. If you're under a lot of stress, your body won't respond properly to the flu shot. Studies show that chronic stress works against your immune system. Find ways to deal with your anxieties. Try some light exercise, find someone to talk with about your problems, or just meditate. Maybe even take a stress management class. Remember, reducing your stress might reduce your chances of getting the flu.

Be a cautious traveler. Unlike the United States, countries in the Southern hemisphere suffer their flu season from April to September. In some tropical areas, flu season is year-round. But even if you're not visiting these places, others in your tour group or on your plane or cruise ship could infect you. Experts advise getting a flu shot before you travel. If the current vaccine is not yet available, ask your doctor about antiviral medication you can take with you in case you get sick on your trip.

Colon cancer

Smart choices help beat this deadly disease

Colorectal cancer often begins quietly, with constipation as its only symptom – but don't underestimate it. This deadly disease is the second leading cancer killer in the United States, and the third most common cancer.

Most cases of colorectal cancer begin with the growth of polyps in the colon. Polyps are common, especially in older people, but they are not always cancerous. Nevertheless, researchers estimate that up to 80 percent of colon cancer deaths could be prevented by removing precancerous polyps quickly.

Since symptoms aren't always noticed early, screening for colon cancer is very important, especially if you're at high risk. Risk factors include a family or personal history of the disease; having a colon or bowel disorder, such as irritable bowel syndrome or colitis; having had ovarian, endometrial, or breast cancer; and eating a diet high in animal fat and low in fiber.

Your chances of getting colorectal cancer also increase as you age. Many cancer organizations recommend regular screening after age 50 and making these changes in your lifestyle.

Eat a high-fiber, low-fat diet. Several recent studies have found no evidence that a high intake of fruits, vegetables, and fiber reduces the occurrence of colon polyps in people who already have polyps. However, the studies lasted only a few years, and they may not have been long enough for the protective effect of diet to show up. The bulk of evidence still suggests that a diet low in fat and high in fruits, vegetables, and fiber can reduce your risk of colon cancer, as well as other diseases, such as heart disease, diabetes, high blood pressure, and obesity.

Choose colorful foods. Eating plenty of fruits and vegetables is important to a healthy diet, and when it comes to cancer prevention, color may be the key. A recent study found that fruits and vegetables containing lutein, a kind of carotenoid, may help prevent colon cancer. Carotenoids are substances that give fruits and vegetables their color. Foods high in lutein include spinach, tomatoes, corn, broccoli, oranges, green beans, lettuce, and cabbage.

Ask your doctor about aspirin. Daily aspirin therapy might reduce your risk of colon cancer. Unfortunately, one study found that it takes 10 years of regular aspirin use, four to six tablets a week, to significantly reduce your risk. A recent study done on rats suggests that acetaminophen (Tylenol) could block the cancer-causing substances in foods and help prevent colon cancer, but more studies are needed.

Stop smoking. If the possibility of developing lung cancer frightens you, consider the increased risk of the second-highest cancer killer, too. A recent study found that smokers were more likely to have colon polyps than nonsmokers, and their polyps tended to be more aggressive. The good news from the study was that stopping smoking decreased that risk dramatically. Even if you've been smoking most of your life, it's worth the effort to quit. Talk with your doctor about new programs and medications that can help.

Eat wheat to defeat colon cancer

When it comes to heavy hitters against colon cancer, wheat bran is Babe Ruth. Time and time again, wheat bran has knocked colon cancer out of the ballpark. A cup of wheat bran gives you a whopping 25 grams of fiber. This kind of fiber, insoluble fiber, adds bulk to your stool and dilutes the carcinogens in it.

It also speeds your stool through the gastrointestinal tract so it's not hanging around causing trouble. This makes wheat bran good for curing constipation and maintaining a healthy gut, as well as protecting you against cancer. But fiber might not be the only hero.

Wheat bran also has phytic acid, a substance with antioxidant properties that may stop tumors. Those who doubt fiber's anticancer power point to phytic acid as a possible explanation for wheat bran's effectiveness against the development of colon tumors. Whether it's the fiber or the phytic acid, wheat bran works. But don't stop there. These foods also protect you from colon cancer.

Opt for oats and barley. When it comes to roller-coasters, bigger and faster means better. If you want to protect yourself against colon cancer, start thinking this way about your stool.

It's the soluble fiber beta-glucan in oats and barley that may give you this protection. It adds bulk to your stool and hurries it through your large intestine. In fact, a study headed by Dr. Joanne Lupton of Texas A&M University showed that eating barley bran flour increased stool weight by almost 50 grams and slashed transit time by 8 hours.

Beta-glucan slows down the movement of food through your stomach and small intestine. But foods normally spend 10 times longer in your large intestine, which absorbs cancer-causing agents. That means a bulkier, faster-moving stool is less likely to hang around and cause problems.

Oats and barley might also battle colon cancer by changing the tiny organisms in your large bowel. When these organisms react with beta-glucan, scientists think they might produce compounds that protect your colon tissue.

"Take any one of these proposed mechanisms," says Dr. Barbara Schneeman, a researcher with the USDA's Agricultural Research Service and professor of agricultural and environmental sciences at the University of California-Davis.

"By itself, it's not enough to prove a relation between fiber and cancer. It could be, in fact, multiple factors coming together. But you need this stuff for a healthy gut. Don't forget in trying to prevent disease, you're trying to keep your gut healthy as well."

Make room for milk. Here's a new twist on mother's advice to "drink your milk so you'll build strong bones and teeth." Research has shown for years that the calcium and vitamin D in milk products may also help prevent colon cancer, particularly among older women. Calcium and, to a lesser extent, vitamin D has reduced the growth of cancer-causers in laboratory rats and in humans.

Two different studies found that eating and drinking dairy products, or taking a supplement with calcium and vitamin D, could play a part in reducing the risk of colon cancer. In one study, people took a supplement of 1,200 milligrams (mg) of calcium carbonate a day (about the same as three Rolaids tablets) and suffered no negative side effects.

At least one small study has indicated that extra calcium doesn't help prevent colon cancer, but the researchers admitted that all 30 people in the study got plenty of calcium in their diets anyway. You may especially need vitamin D if you live in an area with high levels of air pollution or in a northern climate without much sunlight. That's because less sunshine means lower levels of vitamin D in your bloodstream.

Fight cancer with fruits and veggies. Folic acid, a B vitamin also known as folate, is so important to the health of unborn babies that the Food and Drug Administration has proposed that all bread and grain products be fortified with it. It only makes sense that something so essential for pregnant women is important to your good health, too. Folic acid seems to help "turn cancer genes off," according to researchers at Harvard. On the other hand, as few as two alcoholic beverages a day can increase the chances of colon cancer in men and women. The alcohol gets in the way of folic acid's good effects.

Many of the foods you already enjoy contain folic acid, including broccoli, spinach, collards, oranges, lemons, grapefruit, beans, and whole-grain breads and cereals.

Constipation

Prevent 'irregularity' with regular habits

Do you want to stay regular, stop using laxatives, and avoid hemorrhoids? Then follow this action plan to keep your intestines working smoothly.

Get your fill of fiber. Here's how – eat a bowl of wheat bran cereal in the morning, make your lunch sandwich out of whole-grain wheat bread and eat several vegetables at lunch and dinner, or as snacks throughout the day.

That way, you'll get your fill of "insoluble fiber," the kind that works best to prevent constipation. Fiber is the indigestible part of plants. The insoluble type of fiber doesn't dissolve in water. When you eat it, the fiber enters your intestines and holds water there. The water makes your stool soft, bulky, and easy to eliminate. And, since you don't digest fiber, the food goes through your system much more quickly.

You'll find the most insoluble fiber in wheat bran, vegetables, and whole-grain wheat breads and cereals. The cheapest and probably best source of insoluble fiber is raw, unprocessed wheat bran, which is one of the few high-fiber foods that really does call to mind those ugly images of rough, gritty, tasteless foods. But you can easily cover it up by mixing it with your cereal, hot or cold, or baking it into low-fat muffins or breads. It also adds an interesting texture to thick soups and stews.

Psyllium is the type of fiber you find in many bulk laxatives and bran supplements. It's a soluble fiber, which means it dissolves in water and lowers cholesterol, but it's an oddity. The bacteria in your stomach don't break it down as quickly as other soluble fibers, so it also works like an insoluble fiber to increase stool bulk and prevent constipation. A good food source of psyllium is Kellogg's Bran Buds.

Add about 10 grams of fiber to your diet a day until you regularly eat 20 to 35 grams of fiber daily. Take care to introduce extra fiber into your diet gradually. Adding too much fiber too quickly could cause more constipation, gas, and bloating. Make sure you drink plenty of water as you increase the amount of fiber. If you don't, the fiber may just make the problem worse.

Aim for six to eight glasses of liquids a day. Caffeine and alcohol don't count because they cause you to lose water. You need enough water in your body to help keep your stools soft, so you can pass them easily.

Exercise regularly. You should spend at least 20 to 30 minutes three times a week walking or engaging in some other aerobic exercise that you enjoy. Regular exercise helps move food through your intestines faster.

Cheese and constipation may not go hand in hand after all. In a recent study of 21 people ages 68 to 87, researchers found that not one of the study participants complained of constipation or excessive gas even after eating 10 times as much cheese as they normally did. So feel free to enjoy some cheese.

Go when you gotta go. You should go to the bathroom as soon as you feel the urge to have a bowel movement. Constantly ignoring the urge can often lead to hardened stools and uncomfortable constipation.

Get on a schedule. Pick a convenient time, about 10 to 60 minutes after one of your regular meals, to spend about 10 minutes in the bathroom. Go to the bathroom every day after the same meal. Many people find that after breakfast works well. If nothing happens right away, don't worry and don't strain. After a while, your bowels will catch on.

Keep a step stool in your bathroom. Some people find that propping their feet on a footrest during bathroom visits makes bowel movements easier.

Check your medicine cabinet. Ask your doctor if any of the medicines you're taking could cause constipation. Some common culprits include antidepressants, antihistamines, antiparkinsonism drugs, diuretics, and antacids that contain calcium or aluminum. Your doctor may be able to recommend an alternative that's easier on your intestines.

Depression

Beat the blahs with good nutrition

"It's very hard to explain how low you can get," says Lawrence Black. Over 10 years ago, Black, a native of Pennsylvania, began to suffer from depression. The illness came on gradually over time, and Black tried at first to deal with it on his own. Then one night, he woke up and realized he wasn't getting better. "I just couldn't take it anymore," he explains. "It was like I hit a wall."

Black is not alone. Every day depression and other mental illnesses darken the lives of over 340 million people worldwide. Depression brings with it feelings of sadness, pessimism, tiredness, and worthlessness that can last two weeks, two months, or a lifetime.

Everyday activities you once enjoyed and did easily become impossible and joyless. "You get so low, you look for an escape," Black says. For Black, his escape was sleeping and being alone. For others, it might be never sleeping, overeating, alcohol abuse, or even suicide.

Experts aren't sure what's exactly at the root of this tragic mental illness. Problems with the brain's chemistry, genetics, seasonal changes, a recent bout with serious illness, a stressful life situation, like divorce or pregnancy, can bring on depression by themselves or in combination. For Black, it was the death of his father and the illness of his friend and business partner. "They were the two main events that brought the depression on," he believes.

Whatever the cause of deep sadness, you can't just "snap out of it," just like a diabetic can't snap his fingers and get better. If you are depressed, you need to find help. Without it, severe depression will continue to cause serious psychological and even physical damage. Fortunately, Black turned to his wife for support. Together they saw a psychiatrist. It was a tough road to recovery at first. But after try-ing three medications, he and his doctor found one that worked. "It makes me feel," he says, "like I did before – normal."

You can learn a lesson from Black's story – get help. It can work if you are seriously depressed or even if you just have the everyday "blues." Talk with your spouse or other loved ones, join a support group, meditate, start a hobby, pray, exercise – all these activities can help you feel better.

And surprisingly, eating the right foods and focusing on good nutrition can lift your spirits and brighten your day, too.

B vitamins. Believe it or not, a sweet potato or a spinach salad might help you beat the blues. Both are rich in folate and vitamin B6 or pyridoxine. Deficiencies in these two B vitamins can actually bring on the symptoms of depression. Vitamin B6 works by keep-ing your brain's neurotransmitters in balance. These chemicals control whether you feel depressed, anxious, or on a steady keel.

Experts aren't sure why folate fights the "blahs." But they do know low folate levels in your body can deepen depression, and high folate levels can help defeat it. You can find folate in most fruits and vegetables, especially spinach, asparagus, avocados, green peas, and pinto beans.

Eat chicken, liver, and other meats to feed your brain vitamin B6. Plant sources of the vitamin include navy beans, sweet potatoes, spinach, and bananas.

Depression can also signal a deficiency in thiamin, also known as vitamin B1. Stick with whole wheat breads, meats, black beans, and watermelon to raise your thiamin levels. These foods might help you feel more clearheaded and energetic.

Iron. Beating the blues might be as easy as eating iron-rich foods if you have iron-deficiency anemia. Over 2 billion people suffer from this condition and even more live with a less-serious form of iron deficiency. A sour mood is a major symptom of a lack of iron. Other symptoms include pale skin, sluggishness, and having trouble concentrating.

Iron-deficiency anemia often attacks pre-menopausal women, people who regularly take nonsteroidal anti-inflammatory drugs (NSAIDs), and others at risk for chronic blood loss. It's a good idea to visit your doctor if you suspect you're anemic.

To get more iron in your diet, try meat for starters. The darker the cut, the more iron it has. If you're a vegetarian, stick with legumes, fortified cereals, quinoa, and kale – as well as other green leafy vegetables. And it's a good idea to top these foods with a rich source of vitamin C, like lemon juice. The vitamin C will help your body absorb the iron.

Selenium. You probably heard selenium fights cancer, but you might not know the mineral banishes bad moods, too. People who don't eat enough selenium-rich foods tend to be grumpier than people with a high dietary intake, according to recent research. Eat some high-test selenium foods – like seafood, poultry, mushrooms, sea vegetables, and wheat – and feel the effects for yourself.

Carbohydrates. If stress gets you down, a carbohydrate-rich diet might be just what the doctor ordered. Eating mostly carbohydrates during the day, suggests a European study, may make stressful situations more bearable for some people. The scientists fed people either a diet high in carbs and low in protein, or vice versa. Then the scientists put the subjects through a difficult mathematical task. The carbohydrate-rich diet worked to lower stress and depression in some of the subjects.

The carbohydrate diet appears to work by raising the level of tryptophan in your brain. Tryptophan is the amino acid your body needs to make serotonin, the "happy" neurotransmitter.

It's important to remember not all carbohydrates are equal. Nutritionally speaking, carbohydrates from fruits, vegetables, and whole grains and cereals are best. They'll save you from stress and boost your levels of vitamins, minerals, and fiber.

Cast off depression with fish oil

Don't be offended if someone calls you a fathead. You're in good company. Albert Einstein, Thomas Edison, Sir Isaac Newton, and Confucius can be called fatheads, too. That's because fat makes up about 60 percent of the human brain. But you do have a choice over what type of fathead you want to be. You can keep your brain running smoothly with the right kinds of fats or you can gum up the works with too much of the wrong kind. It all depends on what you eat.

Sound fishy? As a matter of fact, it is. The essential fats found in seafood, called omega-3 fatty acids, play a major role in brain function. They may even boost your mood. You need them but can't make them on your own. "Essential fatty acids only appear through your diet," says Dr. William Lands of the National Institutes of Health. That means the next time you're feeling blue, dip into the deep blue sea for a delicious dinner. New medical evidence suggests the omega-3 fatty acids found in fish – called docosahexaenoic acid (DHA) and eicosapentaenoic acid (EPA) – can help drive away depression.

Dr. Andrew Stoll, a Harvard psychiatrist, found that fish oil capsules helped people with bipolar disorder, or manic depression, who go through periods of extreme highs and lows. He says, "The striking difference in relapse rates and response appeared to be highly clinically significant." Stoll suggests the omega-3 fatty acid in fish oil may slow down neurons in your brain, much like the drug Lithium, which is often used to treat manic depression.

Another research group from England noticed that depressed people had less omega-3 fatty acids in their red blood cells than healthy people. It seemed the more severe the depression, the less omega-3.

There is even evidence that EPA can help treat people with schizophrenia, a serious mental illness that can cause delusions, hallucinations, and disorganized behavior.

Some experts believe fish fights depression because neurotransmitters, the brain's Pony Express riders that carry messages from cell to cell, have an easier time wriggling through fat membranes made of fluid omega-3 than any other kind of fat. This means your brain's important messages get delivered.

Fish also has an effect on serotonin levels, one of your brain's good-news messengers. If you don't have enough serotonin, you're more likely to be depressed, violent, and suicidal. If you have low levels of DHA, you also have low levels of serotonin.

More DHA means more serotonin. Most antidepressants, including Prozac, raise brain levels of serotonin. You might be doing the same thing just by eating fish. In other words, gills may be as good as pills.

Whether you're depressed or not, work more omega-3 into your diet and perhaps cut down on omega-6, another type of essential fatty acid found in vegetable oils, meat, milk, and eggs.

Right now, the typical American eats at least 10 times more omega-6 than omega-3, or a ratio of 10-to-1. Some diets push that ratio to 25-to-1 or even higher. Eating fewer fruits, vegetables, and fish and more grain, farm-raised meat, and processed foods puts the omega-6 to omega-3 ratio out of whack.

Not that omega-6 is bad, but too much leads to excess signaling in your brain. Fortunately, omega-3 can help stop the crazy antics of omega-6 and bring things back to normal.

To fix your balance of omega-6 and omega-3, the obvious first step is to eat more fish. Fatty fish, like salmon, herring, mackerel, and tuna, offer the most omega-3, but all seafood contains some. Aim for at least two fatty fish meals per week.

If you're an absolute landlubber who can't stand fish, get some omega-3s from flaxseed and walnuts. Other good sources include dark green, leafy vegetables, like collards, spinach, arugula, kale, and Swiss chard. Remember, the omega-3 in these foods is in the form of alpha-linolenic acid, which the brain can convert to DHA only in small amounts. To get the good stuff your brain prefers, the pre-formed DHA and EPA, you still need to eat fish.

You might also want to consider taking fish oil supplements, which are available in health food stores, pharmacies, and supermarkets. Just one caution – if you're taking blood thinners, check with your doctor before taking these supplements because omega-3s also have blood-thinning effects.

Just as important to your fatty acid balance are the things not to eat, namely soybean and corn oils, both much too high in omega-6 and too low in omega-3. Eliminate all deep-fried foods and margarine and salad dressings that contain corn or soybean oil. Canola oil, which has a more favorable 2-to-1 ratio of omega-6 to omega-3, or olive oil, a monounsaturated oil with the least amount of omega-6, can do wonders for your essential fatty acid balance.

It all boils down to this – the type of fat you eat determines how your brain works. Moreover, your food determines your mood. By getting more omega-3 and less omega-6 into your diet, you can rev your brain, and your spirits, into high gear. And that's no fish story.

Drug-free ways to feel like yourself again

It's a fact of life. Most people get depressed every once in a while. The good news is a long-term study has revealed new ways to treat depression without dangerous drugs.

Enjoy family and friends. Don't just count the number of family members and friends you have – really connect with them. People who are depressed tend to isolate themselves. Stay in touch with your friends and the people you love.

Find meaning in your life. A study conducted by the Northern Arizona University Department of Nursing found that seniors living in retirement communities were less depressed if they had a feeling of purpose and importance that went beyond themselves. A great way to start is by reaching out and helping other people. And learning to appreciate all of the good things in your life is another way to lift your spirits.

Work on staying healthy. People who feel good are less depressed. You'll feel better if you eat well-balanced, healthy meals; get enough sleep; and exercise every day. Most kinds of physical activity reduce stress, get you out of the house, raise your energy level, encourage you to interact with others, and get your mind off your problems.

Numerous studies show that people who exercise regularly are less likely to become depressed than people who don't. Exercise actually stimulates the production of dopamine and serotonin, chemicals in your brain that improve your mood. In fact, for some people, it's just as effective as taking antidepressants and getting counseling. In almost all cases, when people add an exercise program to their drug or counseling treatment, their conditions improve more rapidly and significantly.

Your doctor may prescribe exercise instead of antidepressants. Although the drugs will often bring about a more immediate improvement, in the long run, working out is just as powerful.

Wake up to the light. Depression can affect your sleep. Perhaps you're sleeping too much, or you can't sleep at all. Maybe you wake up several times during the night. When you're tired and have no energy, you feel even more depressed.

These symptoms could mean your internal clock is not running as smoothly as it should. When you adjust your body clock, you adjust your mood. It's easy to do. Simply control the amount and quality of sleep you get each night and how much light you are exposed to at different times of the day.

Even normal levels of indoor, artificial lighting can affect your internal clock. In the evening, dim the lights before winding down. Make your bedroom dark while you sleep. Change your sleep pattern so you are awake in the morning. Open your curtains or blinds. Morning sunshine increases the level of melatonin in your body, a hormone that helps regulate your sleep cycle naturally.

You will sleep better at night and wake up feeling more rested and less depressed if you soak up bright light for several hours every day. But don't use ultraviolet (UV) light because experts aren't sure of its safety. The brighter the light and the longer you are exposed, the more helpful it is in treating depression.

Use your sense of smell. Aromatherapy can help treat many physical and emotional problems, from headaches to depression. Researchers have found that vapors in essential oils trigger a specific part of your brain to release chemicals, such as serotonin, into your nervous system. These brain chemicals help relieve depression by calming you or helping you sleep. Many hospitals are using aromatherapy to reduce stress and encourage good sleep patterns in their patients.

In a recent study at the University of Miami School of Medicine, researchers found that just three minutes of aromatherapy with lavender oil were not only relaxing but relieved depression, as well. To fight the blues, surround yourself with juniper, marjoram, melissa, or orange blossom. You can add them to your bath; massage with them; use a diffuser, vaporizer, candles, aroma lamps, or potpourri burners; spray them in the air; or inhale them straight from the bottle.

Find healing with herbs. In a study of about 300 people, researchers concluded that St. John's wort was just as effective as one of the leading antidepressants in improving quality of life, both emotionally and physically. This is great news because herbal supplements have fewer and less severe side effects than most antidepressants. That means people are more likely to continue taking the supplement.

St. John's wort is a good, safe choice for mild to moderate depression but not severe depression, manic-depression, or obsessive-compulsive disorder.

If you want to use herbs to treat your depression, ask your doctor for advice. Don't stop taking any medicine he prescribed without his approval, and continue seeing him regularly so he can monitor your depression.

Beyond the blues

Sometimes events in your life make you feel blue. Some situational sadness is normal, but if you can't snap out of the depression, or if you feel depressed for no apparent reason, you may be in trouble. And you won't be alone. The National Institute of Mental Health (NIMH) estimates that more than 9 million Americans suffer from clinical depression.

To help you distinguish between just feeling blue and being clinically depressed, check out these symptoms of depression listed by the NIMH.

◆ Persistent sad, anxious, or "empty" mood

◆ Feelings of hopelessness, pessimism

◆ Feelings of guilt, worthlessness, helplessness

◆ Loss of interest or pleasure in hobbies and activities that were once enjoyed, including sex

◆ Insomnia, early-morning awakening, or oversleeping

◆ Loss of appetite and weight loss, or overeating and weight gain

◆ Decreased energy, fatigue, being "slowed down"

◆ Thoughts of death or suicide, suicide attempts

◆ Restlessness, irritability

◆ Difficulty concentrating, remembering, making decisions

◆ Persistent physical symptoms that do not respond to treatment, like headaches, digestive disorders, and chronic pain

If these symptoms sound familiar, you could be suffering from serious depression. See your doctor for a complete checkup to rule out physical problems, then ask him to refer you for professional help.

Diabetes

Survival guide for diabetics

Food choices have changed a lot in the last 100 years. Instead of eating grains and vegetables from old McDonald's farm, you're more likely to drive through McDonald's for a high-fat, low-fiber meal with way too many calories.

You have much more to choose from than your ancestors did, but many of those choices are unhealthy. Today's typical diet will make you overweight, but its lack of fiber-rich carbohydrates can make you feel hungry soon after eating. Worst of all, it can put you at risk for diabetes and heart disease.

Diabetes has become an epidemic in modern countries. About 16 million Americans have this blood sugar disorder that is divided into two categories – type 1 and type 2. Type 1, an autoimmune disease, usually attacks people under the age of 30 and has nothing to do with being overweight.

But type 2, formerly called noninsulin-dependent, accounts for 90 to 95 percent of all cases. This form of diabetes stalks overweight, inactive people. Once a disease of the elderly, type 2 diabetes now appears even in overweight children.

If you have type 2 diabetes, your body probably makes enough insulin but has "forgotten" how to use it. Your cells have become resistant to insulin, so the glucose from the food you eat builds up in your blood instead of nourishing your cells.

High blood sugar levels can start an avalanche of problems, including high cholesterol and high blood pressure. Type 2 diabetics risk blindness, amputations, heart disease, strokes, and nerve damage. Remember, just because it's called "noninsulin-dependent" doesn't mean you'll never need insulin. Many people require insulin after several years with the disease.

If you want to avoid being a victim, you'll have to rethink your diet. Healthy food choices can keep both your weight and blood sugar down. And regular exercise, like brisk walking, will go a long way toward keeping you fit. Even if you already have diabetes, a sensible diet can keep you from developing more health problems. Just make sure you check with your doctor before making any changes to your diet or exercise program.

Here are some simple things you can do to fight diabetes and lower your risk of complications.

High-fiber foods. Fiber helps prevent diabetes because it slows down the process of converting carbohydrates into glucose, says Diana H. Noren, R.D., a certified diabetes counselor in Georgia.

Also, if you eat a high-fiber carbohydrate, your body will respond with less insulin than it would if you eat a low-fiber food, she says. This is better for your overall health because high insulin levels could lead to weight gain and high blood pressure, among other health problems.

In a study of nearly 36,000 women in Iowa, the ones who ate several servings of high-fiber foods every day had a significantly lower risk of developing diabetes than the women who ate little fiber.

Cereals are especially good at warding off diabetes. The women in the study who ate more than 7 grams of cereal fiber a day were 36 percent less likely to become diabetic than women who ate less than half that amount. And 7 grams is not a lot of fiber. A one-cup serving of bran flakes will give you more than 8 grams of cereal fiber. Noren says you can actually eat a little more of a cereal that's high in fiber without harming your total carbohydrate count.

The following foods are high in fiber. Adding them to your diet can help you control your diabetes:

- Oats. A good source of cereal fiber, oats contain a substance called beta glucan that breaks down slowly in your digestive tract. And longer digestion time means lower blood sugar for you. Start your day with a bowl of old-fashioned oatmeal sweetened with a handful of raisins.

- Legumes. Use legumes in soups, casseroles, and salads and cut back on meat. You'll lower your fat intake and increase your fiber at the same time. Legumes can fill you up and help keep you satisfied.

- Figs. The American Diabetes Association recommends figs for a high-fiber treat that can satisfy your sweet tooth, too.

Cornstarch. More than just a thickener for gravy, cornstarch may help control blood-sugar levels and keep you from having an attack of hypoglycemia. This starch is digested and absorbed slowly so it's especially effective for type-1 diabetics prone to low blood glucose levels overnight.

Researchers found that diabetics who drank a mixture of uncooked cornstarch dissolved in a drink without added sugar, such as milk or sugar-free soda, had fewer problems with low blood sugar in the morning. If you have this problem, talk with your doctor about trying this natural solution.

You can also look for snack bars that contain sucrose, protein, and cornstarch. These ingredients release glucose at different speeds, giving you both immediate and long-term help for low blood sugar.

Omega-3 fatty acids. These essential fats all but disappeared when food became mass-produced. Most of the oils used today, like corn, peanut, sesame, and safflower, are high in omega-6 fatty acids. While these fats are essential for good health, if eaten without omega-3s, your immune system can break down.

Researchers have shown that you need omega-3 fats to process insulin. Without them, you run the risk of not using your insulin properly. Insulin resistance often leads to diabetes.

You can find omega-3s in fatty fish, like salmon and mackerel, along with walnuts and flaxseed. And inexpensive canola oil has a good blend of both omega-3 and omega-6 fats. Try eating fatty fish three times a week, and use canola oil for cooking. You can top salads with flaxseed oil, but you can't cook with it.

Cod liver oil. One oil that has high amounts of omega-3 is cod liver oil. Norwegians eat lots of it because they have so little sunlight, and they need the vitamin D found in the oil. A recent study in that country revealed that women who took cod liver oil during pregnancy reduced their child's risk of type 1 diabetes by more than 60 percent. Researchers think the omega-3 fats and vitamin D, either separately or combined, might be responsible for the lower risk.

Vinegar. Add red wine vinegar to your salads, and you can easily slow down the digestion of your meal. Because acidic foods are digested slowly, three teaspoons of vinegar can lower your blood sugar after a meal by as much as 30 percent. Lemon juice works well, too. Try squeezing a fresh lemon into water for a refreshing and healthful drink.

Chromium. Research shows that not getting enough chromium in your diet can make diabetes worse. That's because chromium helps your body process sugar. In the United States, many people don't get enough of this important mineral. Good sources include oysters, liver, whole grains, eggs, cheese, black pepper, potatoes with skin, and nuts.

Biotin. This B-vitamin helps you digest fats and carbohydrates, which are important for diabetics. A deficiency can cause hair loss, rash, loss of appetite, depression, and a swollen tongue. But biotin is easy to get in a healthy diet. Good sources are peanut butter, liver, eggs, cereals, nuts, and legumes.

Vitamin C. Add an orange or grapefruit to your lunch. Research shows the antioxidants in vitamin C could keep you from developing problems with blood sugar. And if you already have diabetes, the acid in the fruit helps slow digestion, keeping your blood sugar more stable.

Get to the 'heart' of diabetes prevention

Most people with diabetes die from some form of heart disease. In fact, the American Heart Association (AHA) says the relationship between these two conditions is so important they consider diabetes a cardiovascular disease.

The good news is you can take steps to protect yourself – if you know the risk factors and what to do about them.

Get tough on cholesterol. Even if your cholesterol numbers fall within the healthy range, you can't relax. The American Diabetes Association (ADA) suggests you keep your bad LDL cholesterol under 100 milligrams per deciliter (mg/dl) and your good HDL cholesterol above 45 mg/dl for men and 55 mg/dl for women.

These guidelines are tougher than those recommended for the general population. Yet research proves if you work hard to lower your LDL cholesterol, you'll reduce your risk of heart disease complications. Get those cholesterol numbers in line with exercise and a healthy diet featuring plenty of fruits, vegetables, and whole grains. Cut back on meat and other sources of saturated fat.

A secret weapon in this battle might be tomato juice. In a clinical study, drinking about two glasses a day for a month kept cholesterol from oxidizing and attaching to your artery walls, a process that hardens and blocks your arteries. In addition, this amount of tomato juice nearly tripled levels of lycopene, a carotenoid proven to guard against heart attacks.

Downsize. Carrying a spare tire in your trunk means you're prepared for an emergency. Unfortunately, carrying a spare tire around your middle means you're at risk for one. Of course, obesity is a classic and deadly risk factor for both heart disease and stroke. In addition, too much fat in the belly can make your liver produce too much glucose. This will throw off how your body processes sugar and can lead to insulin resistance, an early sign of diabetes. Since 80 percent of type 2 diabetics are overweight, this should alert many people.

Luckily, the solution is simple – exercise. And it helps diabetics in many ways. You'll lose weight, improve your blood sugar, and lower your blood pressure and cholesterol. A brisk, 30-minute walk each day can do the trick.

Even if you maintain a healthy weight, exercise is still important. A recent study measuring the fitness of men with type 2 diabetes found that unfit men were twice as likely to die from any cause, including heart disease, as fit men. Not surprisingly, being physically fit helped normal weight diabetics just as much as diabetics who were overweight.

Reduce the pressure. If you're diabetic, your risk for high blood pressure doubles. When you have high blood pressure, your heart must work extra hard to pump blood through your body. The strain leads to heart disease. In fact, high blood pressure might cause up to 75 percent of all cardiovascular disease in diabetics.

Exercising regularly and avoiding foods high in saturated fat – like meat, egg yolks, whole milk, butter, and cheese – and high in fruits, vegetables, and whole grains, can help keep your blood pressure under control.

But to get your blood pressure down to the ADA's target of less than 130/80, you might need medication. The American Heart Association thinks ACE (angiotensin converting enzyme) inhibitors are the best choice in blood pressure lowering drugs. Research shows they not only lower blood pressure, but also cut down on kidney disease.

While ACE inhibitors could be your first choice of medication, they're not for everyone. Even if they help, many times you need more than one medication to get your blood pressure down to a safe level. Beta-blockers and diuretics are among other effective options. Work with your doctor to find what's best for you.

Give up the cigarettes and alcohol. Two easy ways to lower your risk for heart disease – and other health problems – are to quit smoking and cut down on drinking. Health experts warn against drinking more than two drinks a day for men, and one for women. One drink equals 5 ounces of wine, a 1-1/2-ounce shot of 80-proof spirits, or 12 ounces of beer.

Look in unexpected places. Traditional risk factors, like the ones listed earlier, don't entirely explain why people with diabetes are more at risk for heart disease. The answer might lie in your blood. Researchers conducting the Atherosclerosis Risk in Communities (ARIC) study found that low levels of a protein called albumin and high levels of several blood clotting substances, as well as white blood cells, increased the likelihood of heart disease in diabetics. All of these things can indicate inflammation or problems with the cells lining your blood vessels and heart.

Your action plan might be as simple as taking an aspirin a day. The ADA already recommends aspirin for all diabetics because it keeps your blood from clotting. Because aspirin has anti-inflammatory powers, it might be just the thing to protect diabetics from heart disease. Aspirin also helps protect your eyes from diabetic retinopathy. Just remember to check with your doctor before starting aspirin therapy.

Fetch help for low blood sugar

Get ready to unleash a powerful new weapon in your battle with diabetes. This weapon alerts you when your blood sugar is low, and brings you your slippers.

According to a recent article in the *British Medical Journal*, dogs have displayed odd behavior during their owners' hypoglycemic episodes. Most surprising, the dogs signaled something was wrong even before their owners realized their blood sugar was low. In some cases, dogs have probably saved lives by waking their owners in the night.

How dogs can sense low blood sugar is a mystery. But if you have a dog, pay attention to any strange behavior. You just might be receiving some kind of canine communication.

If you don't have a dog, but you have trouble recognizing the signs of hypoglycemia, experience nighttime episodes, and live alone, consider a pound puppy. Man's best friend might also be your best protection.

Heel to toe foot care

One out of every 170 diabetics will have a foot amputated due to the nerve disorder peripheral neuropathy. Horrifying statistics considering you can prevent this tragic outcome with good foot care. About a third of all diabetics suffer from neuropathy, which can cause special problems for your feet.

Because this disorder damages your nerves, you may not feel pain from injuries or irritations. You are more likely to develop ulcers or infections, and your foot shape can actually change. So it's critical that you pay special attention to your shoes and feet.

The first step to better foot care is scheduling a thorough foot exam with your doctor at least once a year. However, if a problem arises between visits, don't wait – see your doctor right away.

Whether you see a general practitioner, a diabetes specialist, or a podiatrist, make sure he tests the nerve function and circulation in your feet. He should also check your skin and nails and take care of any routine maintenance you can't manage yourself. Talk about changes you've noticed. Do your feet feel different? Are they a different shape or color? Then, each day, do everything you can to prevent a minor problem from becoming a major pain.

Examine your feet every day. Look for blisters, cuts, scrapes, sores, redness, bruises, infections, swelling, or bumps. Get someone to help you, or use a mirror if you can't see the bottoms of your feet.

Wash with mild soap. Use warm water (check the temperature with your wrist) and don't soak – that removes calluses that can protect sensitive spots. Dry your feet carefully, especially between your toes.

Treat dry skin. If your feet seem especially dry, check with your doctor to make sure you don't have athlete's foot, which needs special care. If it's just dry skin, apply a small amount of petroleum jelly or lotion before you put on your socks and shoes. (Most people don't need expensive specialty products.) This will keep your skin from cracking. But make sure you avoid moisturizing the skin between your toes.

Sock it to 'em. Wear socks that are soft and thick enough for extra protection. Choose material that will draw moisture away from your skin, like acrylic. Avoid cotton, which stays wet; thin, slippery socks or stockings; and socks that have holes or seams.

Choose shoes with care. They should fit well, even over your thickest socks, with enough room so your toes don't rub. Take any inserts with you when you go shopping to ensure a fool-proof fit. Don't assume you take the same size you've worn for years, since your foot may become wider and flatter. If necessary, visit a pedorthist, a corrective shoe specialist.

Look before you lace. Before putting on your shoes, check inside for pebbles or other objects, and make sure your shoes don't have holes or tears that could cause injury.

Never go barefoot outside. Be careful indoors, too. Keep slippers by your bed to avoid bumping into things at night.

Take special care of your toenails. Cut them straight across, but file down sharp corners that might cut the next toe. If you develop a nail fungal infection, don't use an over-the-counter remedy without talking with your doctor first. He might want to prescribe an oral medication, which seems to be more effective.

Smooth out the rough spots. Use a dry towel or pumice stone to rub away dead skin.

Stay away from self-surgery. Don't cut off corns, calluses, or warts yourself, and never use nonprescription remedies to remove them. The harsh chemicals can damage the surrounding healthy tissue. Take these problems to your doctor.

Sleep tight tonight. Don't use hot water bottles or heating pads to warm your feet at night. Wear socks instead. If the bedcovers are irritating or heavy on your feet, buy a special hoop from a medical supply store that holds the sheet off your legs.

Get your blood moving. Try not to cross your legs when you sit. This keeps the blood from flowing freely to your legs and feet. Exercise will also improve circulation.

10 conditions you can fight with fiber

Bumping up the fiber in your diet can help you avoid these conditions — or deal with them in a healthier way.

◆ Diabetes. Fiber helps improve the way your body handles insulin and glucose.

◆ Heart attacks and strokes. Soluble fiber helps eliminate much of the cholesterol that can clog your arteries.

◆ Constipation and hemorrhoids. Fiber keeps the stool moist, soft, and easy to eliminate.

◆ Appendicitis. A soft bowel content can help protect you from appendicitis.

◆ Diverticulosis. As your body processes fibrous foods, it tones up your intestinal muscles. This helps prevent pouches, called diverticula, which can cause abdominal pain if they become inflamed.

◆ Weight gain. When you eat bulky, fiber-rich foods like vegetables and grains, you leave less room for fat. And since the fiber swells, you'll feel satisfied faster.

◆ Impotence. Fiber helps maintain strong blood flow to the penis by lowering your cholesterol and keeping your blood vessels unclogged.

◆ Cancer. Fiber speeds cancer-causing compounds out of the digestive system more quickly – before they have a chance to make trouble.

Diarrhea

7 ways to conquer diarrhea

What you choose to eat when you have diarrhea can make a big difference in your recovery – so choose carefully.

Cook up some rice. Want a simple, safe, yet inexpensive treatment? Boil some rice. Scientists have discovered a substance in cooked rice that keeps your intestinal cells from producing too much chloride, which can cause diarrhea. Many underdeveloped countries have been using this remedy for years. They simply drink the cooled water left in the pot after cooking rice. In addition to inhibiting your chloride secretion, this liquid contains starch and nutrients that help rehydrate your body.

Bite into an apple. This juicy fruit can relieve both diarrhea and constipation. Apples contain pectin, a soluble fiber that absorbs water in your stomach and intestines. It swells and forms a gummy mass that moistens and softens the stool to help ease difficult bowel movements. At the same time, the bulk formed by pectin firms up the watery stool of diarrhea, changing it to a thicker consistency.

Drink plenty of liquids. When you have diarrhea, you lose body fluids. It's important to replace the lost water and electrolytes – salts and minerals normally found in your blood, tissue fluids, and cells. Drink at least eight to 10 glasses of liquid each day to replenish your body's fluids. Water, caffeine-free sodas, popsicles, herbal tea, broth, or gelatin are good choices. Or try this recipe – mix one teaspoon of salt and four teaspoons of sugar into one quart of water. Drink two cups of this every hour.

Eat some berries. Dried blueberries are a popular European remedy for diarrhea. If you can't find them at your grocery store, make your own. Simply spread some fresh berries out in the sun until they wrinkle and shrivel up. Then, either eat about three table-spoons of the berries or crush them, boil them for 10 minutes, strain, and drink as a tea. Remember – eating fresh blueberries won't have the same effect. Another choice is the bilberry. It's a variety of blueberry that also works well on diarrhea. You may find dried bilberries or bilberry extract in your local herb shop.

Give the BRAT a try. To ease your digestive system back onto solids after a bout with diarrhea, try the BRAT diet. Instead of moving right from water to normal eating, the BRAT method suggests a transitional diet of Bananas, Rice, Applesauce, and Toast. These foods are both nutritious and gentle on your digestive tract. After things have returned to normal, eat soft, bland foods, such as cooked cereal, rice, eggs, custard, bananas, yogurt, soda crackers, toast, skinless baked potatoes, or chicken for a day or two.

Beware of these grains. Are you suffering from diarrhea after a particular meal? Think about what you just ate. If your menu included wheat, rye, barley, or another grain, you may be allergic to gluten, a mixture of proteins found in these grains. This inherited allergy, called celiac sprue disease, can severely damage the lining of your intestines. If you think this may be causing your problems, try substituting products made with rice, corn, or soybean flour.

Take it slowly. For several days after experiencing diarrhea, stay away from fruit; alcohol; caffeine; milk; gassy foods, like beans, cabbage, and onions; and spicy, greasy, or fatty foods.

Diverticulosis

How to dodge diverticulosis

Chances are, you're going to get diverticulosis. You may even have it now. Half the people over age 60 have the pea-sized pouches along the large intestine walls called diverticula.

But it's not a problem as long as they don't bother you. It's when the diverticula become infected and inflamed that you may begin to regret the diet habits that gave you those pouches. Infected diverticula can cause cramps, pain, tenderness in the left side of your stomach, gas, and blood in your stools. That's called diverticulitis. But you can keep the pouches from growing in the first place by changing your diet to include less fat and red meat and more fiber.

Sacrifice the steak. Many researchers believe red meat causes bacteria in your intestines to weaken your colon and make it easier for diverticula to form. Yet, fish and chicken don't seem to have this effect.

The fat in meat is also a problem. Researchers have found that fat from other sources, like dairy, is much less likely to lead to diverticulosis than fat from red meat. In fact, one study of 50,000 doctors showed that those who ate a lot of fatty meat and not much fiber were most likely to develop diverticulosis. It may be tough to give up those juicy steaks, but doing so will help pave the way for problem-free digestion.

Learn to love grains. Fiber is the biggest key to fighting off diverticulosis because, quite simply, it makes things easy on your colon. Straining during bowel movements is a prime culprit in causing diverticula to form – by pushing out weak spots in the wall of your colon. Fiber softens your stool and keeps the pressure down in your bowels, so things move more smoothly. It also helps stimulate the muscles of your digestive tract, which keeps the walls of your intestines toned and healthy.

The American Dietetic Association says you should eat 20 to 35 grams of fiber every day. The World Health Organization recommends 27 to 40 grams. Grains are possibly the best sources for adding fiber to your diet. Try these fiber powerhouses, but keep in mind, the more a grain is processed, the less benefit you get.

- Bran. The outer husk of grains, or bran, is the greatest source of grain fiber you can eat. You can find bran in everything from cereals and breads to snack foods.

- Barley. This is also a good source of fiber, but keep an eye on what kind you buy. Whole-grain barley has 31 grams of fiber a cup, while pearl barley has only six. Why? Processing.

- Oats. You'll see this grain in many forms, but oat bran is probably your best bet for fiber-packing power. Just one-third of a cup provides 5 grams of fiber.

- Other grains. Experiment with other, less-common grains, such as wild rice, rice bran, rice flour, rye flour, semolina, bulgur, millet, and buckwheat grass. They'll add some pizzazz to your everyday menu.

Enjoy your fruits and veggies. Grains aren't the only name in the high-fiber game. Fruits and vegetables encourage the growth of microbes in your intestines that aid digestion. These microbes keep things "moving along," making it harder for diverticula to form or become infected. Some of your best bets in the fruit category are blackberries (6 grams per cup), raspberries (5 grams), and blueberries (4 grams).

On the vegetable side, beans and peas are your strongest ally. Broad beans are the best (8 grams per cup), followed by lentils, black beans, limas, pintos, baked, kidneys, all the way down to green peas, chickpeas, and black-eyed peas (4 grams).

One thing to remember about fiber – when you add more to your diet, be sure to take it slow. Sudden increases can make you feel bloated and gassy. Also, fiber absorbs a lot of water, and you must replace it or risk dehydration. Guard against this by drinking one-and-a-half to two quarts of water every day.

Keep your diet healthy by filling up on fiber and cutting back on red meat, and your intestines will reward you by staying smooth and inflammation free.

Dry eyes

Simple ways to soothe irritated eyes

The eyes, some say, are the windows to the soul. But when your "windows" feel gritty and scratchy, it can really dull your spirit. Normally, your body bathes your eyes in soothing teardrops. But if you have the condition called dry eyes, you may feel like they are being rubbed with sandpaper instead.

Itchy, red, swollen eyes are probably the symptoms you notice first. You also may be bothered by blurred vision and a burning sensation. A stringy mucus might form in your eyes, and wearing contact lenses can become unbearable.

Tears may not come even when you feel like crying. But, on the other hand, you may find your eyes are watery. This seems a strange symptom of dry eyes, but healthy tears contain oil and mucus. Water alone doesn't coat and cling to your eyes properly. Instead, it evaporates quickly, leaving them unprotected and dry.

You are more likely to experience dry eyes if you:

■ are over 40 – especially if you are a woman who is post-menopausal

■ have allergies

■ wear contact lenses

■ spend a lot of time at the computer

■ do close reading or other detail work

Your dry eyes also could be caused by Sjogren's syndrome, especially if you experience dry mouth as well. This is a serious autoimmune disorder that destroys the glands that produce tears and saliva. In addition to the other symptoms of dry eyes, people with Sjogren's often notice that fluorescent light really bothers them. An eye doctor can test your eyes to determine if this is the cause of your problem.

Fortunately, most of the time dry eyes is a temporary condition. Usually all you need to do is give your eyes a good rest, and they'll be moist and comfortable again. Following these soothing remedies should help put the twinkle back in your eyes.

Avoid irritants from the environment. Try to stay away from smoke, toxic fumes, and other pollutants that can bother your eyes. You may even need to leave off your eye make-up.

Add some moisture. Dry air means dry eyes. So add moisture to the air in your home or office with a humidifier. You'll also find it helpful to drink extra water, especially when flying. Airplane cabins tend to have extra-dry air.

Don't rub it in. It's such a temptation to dig at those itchy eyes, but dry eyes are easily infected. Although it might take some self-control, "hands off" is the best policy.

Protect your peepers. Dry eyes are sensitive to bright light, so wear sunglasses when you go outside. You may even want to wear swim or ski goggles or moisture chamber glasses, especially if Sjogren's syndrome is the cause of your problem. They help to prevent moisture from evaporating as quickly.

Take a break and blink. Do you spend a lot of time reading, using a computer, or doing other close work? You are less likely to blink when performing these tasks, and if you don't, your eyes will suffer. So bat those eyelashes as often as possible.

Use artificial tears. For occasional, short-term use, try tear substitutes. They soothe and protect your eyes just like real tears. But don't use them too often, or they will interrupt your eyes' natural tear production. You should also avoid products with preservatives, which can make the problem worse. Instead of liquid drops, you might prefer to use an ointment. Because it's thicker and stickier, it will stay on the surface of your eye longer. Use ointments at bedtime because they can blur your vision.

You can also get long-lasting soluble inserts. Lacrisert is an example of one without preservatives. You place a tiny pellet inside your lower eyelid where it melts slowly over six to eight hours and helps thicken your tears.

Be careful with contacts. If you wear contact lenses, be especially careful about what you put in your eyes. Drops and ointments may make your eyes more comfortable, but they could mask a serious problem with the contacts themselves.

As a rule, stick with a rewetting solution designed for use with your brand of contacts, or use medications recommended by your eye doctor. In most cases, you'll need to remove the contacts before applying any medication. Follow your doctor's instructions or the package directions about how long to wait before replacing them.

Get some vitamin A. This vitamin is essential for healthy eyes. You'll find it in meat and dairy products. Also, brightly colored fruits and vegetables are high in beta carotene, which converts to vitamin A in your body. You can get vitamin A through supplements, but too much can be dangerous.

Monitor your medications. Dry eyes could be caused by medicines you take. Decongestants, diuretics, general anesthetics, beta-adrenergic blockers, antimuscarinics, and thiabendazole are likely culprits. Talk with your doctor about your situation. Another medication would do just as well without this side effect.

See your doctor often. Regular checkups are important to your eyes' health. And if dry eyes don't clear up quickly or are a chronic problem, you'll need to see your eye doctor more often. You could have damage to the eye or a blocked tear duct that needs treatment by an ophthalmologist.

Dry mouth

Easy-to-swallow tips for dry mouth

Everyone has felt that awful apprehension before a special event that causes your stomach to flutter and your mouth to go dry – nothing is more of a nuisance.

Many prescription or over-the-counter medications also make your mouth feel as dry as the Sahara. Drugs for depression, high blood pressure, pain, weight loss, and flu or cold symptoms can leave you unbearably parched.

Dehydration, heat exhaustion, salty foods, infected salivary glands, diabetes, or simply getting older are all common causes of dry mouth. But if you're a post-menopausal woman over 50 who suddenly finds her mouth and eyes dry, you may be suffering from a condition called Sjogren's (show-grins) syndrome. Health professionals say nine out of 10 sufferers are women.

This is a disease in which your immune system attacks your moisture-producing glands so you don't create as much saliva or tears as you need. It's not a life-threatening condition, but it does get progressively worse, and it can damage your eyes and mouth if the symptoms aren't treated.

Saliva is important to your health because it cleans your mouth of bacteria, helps heal wounds and sores, begins the process of digestion, and keeps your mouth lubricated. Without it, you'll have problems talking and eating, and you may develop painful mouth sores, fungal infections, and tooth decay.

There is no known cure for Sjogren's syndrome, but you can head off problems and ease your symptoms with a little planning and know-how.

Practice good oral hygiene. Brush your teeth, or at least rinse out your mouth, every time you eat. Use a soft toothbrush. Try a device that uses water to irrigate your mouth. Floss regularly but gently. Use home fluoride treatments and fluoride toothpaste. See your dentist more often, maybe three or four times a year, for a checkup, thorough cleaning, and fluoride treatment.

Avoid alcohol, caffeine, and smoking. They dry out your mucous membranes.

Get your juices flowing. Chew sugarless gum (especially those containing the sugar substitute xylitol), drink sugar-free sodas, or suck on hard candy or lemons.

Drink plenty of liquids. Sip throughout the day but especially with meals. This will help moisten your food, making it easier for you to swallow. Milk is a good choice, since it seems to coat and soothe your mouth and can help prevent tooth decay.

Control your air quality. Use a humidifier to moisten the air, and avoid air-conditioning and heated air whenever possible. They are both drying.

Send in a substitute. You can also take advantage of several products designed to substitute for your own saliva. They are the most effective way to moisten a severely parched throat and mouth. Some even contain fluoride to protect your teeth from decay. Look for those products with the American Dental Association seal of approval.

Whether your dry mouth is a result of chronic illness or just a temporary challenge, it can be annoying. But today, more than ever before, you have a variety of ways to make your dry mouth feel normal again.

Dry skin

Shed flaky skin with natural remedies

You know that scaly, itchy, dry sensation that means your skin will soon be molting like a garden snake. You can feel it from your lips to your feet and everywhere in between. Although it happens most often in winter, when indoor air is heated and dry and you tend to use hotter water, it can happen any time.

Whether your irritated skin is from sunburn and swimming, spring cleaning and detergents, or just plain aging, try these tips for soothing relief.

Be cool. Wash your skin with warm or cool water, never hot.

Soak up some softness. Baths are actually less drying to your skin than showers – as long as you use warm water and don't soak longer than 10 minutes.

Take a break. Try to bathe every other day or even just a few times a week. This will reduce how often you strip the protective oils from your skin.

Heat the air, not the water. Warm up your bathroom, with a space heater if necessary, so you'll feel more comfortable bathing in cooler water.

Choose a mild soap. Save the strong, antibacterial deodorant soaps for your underarms, feet, and genital area.

Stop scrubbing. Don't rub your skin too hard after bathing. In fact, patting or blotting with a soft towel is best.

Moisturize. Pat on a lotion right after your bath or shower to lock in moisture.

Avoid the elements. Don't expose your skin to too much sun, wind, or cold.

Go tropical. Avoid dry air if possible. Keep a humidifier running in your home or office.

Balance your diet. Eat plenty of foods containing vitamins A and C to keep your skin smooth and supple. For vitamin A, choose dark green and orange fruits and vegetables, meat, and dairy products. To get extra vitamin C, eat citrus fruits, sweet red peppers, strawberries, and other fruits and vegetables.

Turn on the tap. Drink lots of water every day – at least three large glasses.

Don't forget your fingers. Make it a habit to wear gloves when you do housework or dishes to protect your hands from drying chemicals and hot water.

If you're still not able to beat the dryness or annoying itch, visit a dermatologist. He can prescribe special creams, ointments, or even an oral antihistamine. He'll also try to find out what's causing your problem – allergies, a drug reaction, or some other condition.

Eyestrain

Sharper eyesight without glasses

To transform a weak body into a muscular one, you must exercise faithfully. If you find that you keep replacing your old glasses with stronger ones, perhaps you should give your eyes a good workout as well.

"Just as you can develop your physical fitness," says Dr. Robert-Michael Kaplan, author of *Seeing Without Glasses*, "you can also improve the fitness of your eyes – the way they work together, their stamina, and their interaction with your brain."

Although your vision will tend to weaken with age, Kaplan believes you can take action to slow this inevitable decline. "Your eye muscles can be exercised," he says. "The nerve connection from the brain to your eyes can be stimulated. Blood flow to your eyes can be increased."

You don't need a gym for these vision-training exercises. You can do them wherever you are.

Think to blink. The simple act of blinking moistens your eyes, stretches your eye muscles, massages your eyeballs, and forces your pupils to dilate and contract.

Most people don't blink often enough, especially when reading, driving, watching television, or working at the computer. Kaplan recommends blinking every three seconds.

Practice eye aerobics. Six muscles connect to each of your eyeballs and help them move up and down, side-to-side, and inward and outward. Here's an exercise that can strengthen them and improve the coordination of your eyes.

Sit with your feet firmly on the floor, hands in your lap or supported on the arms of your chair. With your eyes open or closed, face forward. Then take a few deep breaths while relaxing your neck and shoulders.

Stretch your eyes upward as high as they will comfortably go while you breathe in. Hold your breath for a few moments, and then stretch your eyes downward as low as you can without straining as you breathe out. Do this three times.

Next, stretch your eyes sideways to the right, then up to the right. Then stretch down to the left, up to the left, and down to the right. Stay relaxed as you repeat these exercises.

Rest under the palms. After doing the stretching exercises, "cool down" just as you would after any workout. First, warm your palms by rubbing them vigorously together. Lace your fingers together over your forehead with your palms cupped over your eyes, shutting out the light. Rest your eyes in the warm darkness for a few minutes, while taking 20 to 50 deep breaths.

"When you remove your palms," says Kaplan, "you'll observe that colors are much brighter, you'll see more contrast, and you'll enjoy a wonderful relaxed feeling in your eyes and brow muscles." This technique, called palming, is also a good way to take a break from watching television or using the computer.

Soak in sunlight. Kaplan says natural light is good for your eyes. He recommends going outside early in the day, before 10:00 a.m., and late in the afternoon, after 4:00 p.m.

To relax your eyes, close them and face the sun, letting it warm your eyelids. Then turn your head gently from side to side for about five minutes.

Avoid the brightest time of day and never look directly into the sun. When you can't use natural sunlight, you can substitute the light from an incandescent bulb.

See with both sides of your brain. Your eyes alone can't provide you with sight. In fact, as much as 90 percent of what makes it possible to see may take place in your brain.

The right side of your brain controls the left side of your body, including your left eye, and the left side of your brain controls the right side of your body. You need to use both sides to keep your eyes working together.

This exercise, called thumb zapping, is a good way to tell if you are using both sides of your brain. Begin by sitting comfortably in a chair that supports your back. Look steadily at an object 5 to 20 feet away. Slowly bring your thumb into your line of vision, about 8 inches in front of your face. If you are using your eyes together, you will see two thumbs.

If you see only one thumb, or one is clearer than the other, it means you aren't using your eyes equally. Deep breathing, blinking, and palming your eyes can help you strengthen your whole-brain seeing.

Fine-tune your focus. Your ancient ancestors probably had keen eyesight. As hunters and gatherers, they spent most of their time outside, their eyes darting here and there, always on the alert for food or danger. By constantly refocusing close up, a stone's throw away, and into the far distance, they gave their vision a good workout every day.

Today, however, you are more likely to spend your days indoors staring at a flat surface, like the television or computer screen. To avoid couch-potato eyes and improve your focus, try these remarkable exercises.

- Frequently glance away from the screen and quickly bring a distant object into focus.

- Hold out your thumb as in the thumb-zapping exercise. Switch your focus from your thumb to a distant object and back to your thumb again.

■ With neck and shoulders relaxed, practice crossing your eyes. (Don't worry, they won't get stuck.) Focus on your thumb, holding it a few inches in front of your face. Follow it as you bring it close enough to touch your nose. You should feel the muscles pull a little as your eyes turn in.

■ When driving, frequently shift your focus, from on-coming traffic to the dashboard, to the side mirror, to the rear-view mirror. Look to one side of the road and then the other. Read the license plate of the car in front of you, as well as signs at a distance.

In addition to these exercises, Kaplan also has recommendations about nutrition, attitude, and full-body exercise. You can learn more at his Web site <www.beyond2020vision.com>.

Falling

Spring into action to prevent falls

Each year, about one out of three people over the age of 65 falls. The injuries and complications from these falls often result in severe lifestyle changes. Many people are forced into nursing homes after a fall because they can no longer get around and care for themselves. Don't lose your independence because of a preventable accident. Take steps to protect yourself now.

Beware of the stairs. Make sure your stairs have handrails on both sides and use them. Cover your stairs with tight-knit carpeting or nonslip treads. And don't place things on lower steps that you plan to take upstairs later. Keep your stairs completely clutter-free.

Follow the path of least resistance. Arrange your furnishings so there is plenty of room to move freely without having to go around or over obstacles. Keep throw rugs off the beaten path, and tuck all electrical cords safely out of harm's way.

Keep your floors and hallways clean. Wipe up any spills or tracked-in moisture immediately. Don't wax your kitchen floor or the hardwood floor in the hall. Waxed floors are slippery and dangerous. Keep muddy shoes, umbrellas, and other items out of high-traffic areas. They're just waiting to be tripped over.

Let there be light. Be sure your home is well lit, inside and out, particularly in areas of uneven or awkward footing, such as stairs. For security at night, keep a night-light burning in the bathroom, the bedroom, and wherever else you may roam.

Brace yourself in bed and bath. In the bathroom, use nonslip backing on bath mats and rugs. If your tub is slippery, use nonslip tape to help you keep your footing. If you have trouble getting up and down, install a handrail in the tub and next to the toilet. And don't lock your bedroom or bathroom door. If you fall and need help, you want help to be able to get to you.

Keep it down. Don't store things in high places that you need frequently. Whether it's your measuring cups in the kitchen or your favorite books in the family room, keep important items within easy reach. If you have to get something on a high shelf, always use a step stool, never a chair. If possible, get a step stool with handles.

Dress for success. Sensible shoes are a must for good balance. Avoid shoes that are unstable, like high heels and shoes with thick soles. Instead, go for snug, comfortable shoes with rubber soles and laces, and always keep your laces tied.

Get an eye exam. Being able to see also helps you avoid tripping over things. If you need glasses, wear them.

Take your time. Sitting up too fast upon waking, or jumping to your feet before you've had a chance to adjust to the light, can cause head rushes and dizziness. After sitting up in bed, wait for a few seconds on the side of the bed and get your bearings before you stand.

To make this easier, and to avoid injury if you fall off the bed, use a bed that's not too far off the ground. If you can sit on the edge comfortably with your feet on the floor, that's a pretty convenient and safe height for you.

If, after all these precautions, you fall anyway, try to stay calm. Once you've composed yourself, check to see if you're hurt, and if so, how badly. If you can move comfortably, slide yourself to the nearest support – a chair or a wall – and try to stand. If you can't get yourself to your feet, crawl carefully to the phone and call friends or 911 for help.

Fibromyalgia

Fight pain with a personal plan

If you suffer from fibromyalgia, you can learn a lot from Dottie Abbott. A petite, delicate-looking woman in her "golden years," she arrives at tai chi class at the University of West Georgia with a lively step and a friendly smile. You'd never guess she had ever been slowed down by any disease.

But about nine years ago, Dottie had coronary artery bypass surgery. She thinks that was the trigger for the onset of fibromyalgia syndrome (FMS). This disorder, which affects muscles, ligaments and tendons, is not life-threatening. Yet, the symptoms, which include chronic pain and fatigue, can really make life miserable.

Dottie, however, is living proof that life doesn't have to stop when you have FMS. Although there is no cure, with help and self-discipline, you can work out a plan for managing the symptoms. These are some of the things that work for Dottie.

Learn the facts. "If you have fibromyalgia," says Dottie, "the most important thing is to learn all you can about it." This takes away some of the mystery and helps you plan your strategies for dealing with it.

Rita Evans, a licensed clinical social worker who supervises the fibromyalgia self-care program at Dekalb Medical Center in Decatur, Ga., agrees with Dottie on the importance of being informed.

"This condition is not exactly a disease," she explains. "It is a syndrome – a cluster of symptoms. It's hard to diagnose because there is no definitive test. Doctors have to rule out other causes first, so the average diagnosis takes about two years." If you have pain you think might be caused by fibromyalgia, Evans suggests you see a doctor who is a rheumatologist. Since they are the experts in this field, you should be able to get a faster diagnosis.

Build a network of support. Dottie thinks family members also need to learn about fibromyalgia. She says living with this condition can be hard on everybody. It requires the kind of patience that only comes when you know what's going on.

"What people with the syndrome need most," says Evans, "is to be heard and understood. They experience real pain, and they need those around them to affirm that they are sane."

Some people get encouragement from a support group. Since it's estimated that FMS affects 6 million Americans, it shouldn't be hard to find one. Evans says an education-based group that focuses on self-discipline is best. Spending a lot of time talking about feelings isn't very helpful with this syndrome.

Keep moving. Dottie says if she doesn't exercise, her muscles knot up, making movement slow and painful. "I know people with FMS who just sit around and suffer," she says. "But you can't do that or you'll be miserable."

When she first started tai chi classes three years ago, Dottie was having a lot of trouble with her balance. The progress was slow at first, but in time she learned to move freely and confidently and rarely has a problem with balance now.

Dottie practices yoga and finds the deep breathing and stretching help her muscles stay loose. In addition, she walks regularly, every day if the weather is nice. And she lifts light weights and gets two therapeutic massages a week.

Give attention to others. Dottie finds she handles pain better if she doesn't just focus on herself. So she keeps mentally involved in activities in her hometown of Carrollton, Ga. She teaches adult literacy classes as a volunteer two mornings a week. And she's on the board of directors of the League of Women Voters.

Stay calm. Stress can trigger fibromyalgia pain, but Dottie has learned to see it coming and side-step it with relaxation. From time to time when she drives into nearby Atlanta to visit her children, she uses the breathwork she learned from yoga and tai chi. "When I get stuck in traffic," she says, "I just take three deep breaths and relax and let all those other people worry with the frustration. I tell myself everything is just fine."

Get some rest. If you want to stay active in spite of FMS, it's important to get plenty of rest. But that's not easy when you are hurting all over.

Evans says some people find a low dose of an antidepressant – at chronic pain levels, not at clinical depression levels – helps them rest. But Dottie turned down her doctor's offer of drugs. "Everybody handles it differently," she says, "but I think for me exercise takes the place of medication."

"Mild depression often goes with FMS," says Evans. "But touch, exercise, and being with positive people releases endorphins, which relieve depression."

And to round out your self-care plan, Evans recommends eating regular, nutritious meals. As part of an overall healthy lifestyle, these steps, she feels, take the emphasis off FMS symptoms and make it easier to get on with your life.

Gallstones

Easy ways to stay stone free

Horses never have gallstones because, like many animals, they don't have gallbladders. The gallbladder is an organ you can live without, too.

Your gallbladder stores bile, a digestive fluid made by the liver. Sometimes substances in your bile – usually cholesterol – crystallize into gallstones. Some stones don't cause any symptoms. They are called "silent" stones and don't require treatment.

When gallstones grow large or block any of the ducts that carry bile from the liver to the small intestine, they can set off intense pain in your right side or upper abdomen. The pain may also radiate to your right shoulder or between your shoulder blades. These symptoms, which frequently occur after eating or at night, are often mistaken for those of a heart attack, appendicitis, ulcers, or irritable bowel syndrome.

If any of the ducts remain blocked for a significant period of time, severe damage can occur to the gallbladder, liver, and pancreas. Warning signs of a serious problem are constant pain, fever, and jaundice (a yellow tint to your skin or eyes).

Treatment sometimes involves surgically removing the gallstones or the gallbladder. If the gallbladder is removed, bile flows out of the liver and goes directly into the small intestine.

Many health experts say you can avoid painful gallstones by changing your diet and lifestyle. A recent study at the University of Buffalo found that a typical Western lifestyle – too much saturated fat and refined sugar and too little exercise and fiber – increases your risk for gallstones. The lead author Maurizio Trevisan says,

"This study confirms that gallbladder disease is one of the diseases of Western civilization. It is one more message that a diet high in fat and refined sugar and a pattern of low physical activity can get you into all kinds of trouble."

And anyone who has experienced the pain of gallstones can tell you it is definitely trouble. So get busy and make some simple changes in the way you live.

Fiber. Filling up on fiber instead of fat might protect you from gallbladder disease. Vegetarians are less likely to get gallstones, possibly because they eat less saturated fat and more fiber. Fiber increases movement of food through your colon, which could reduce the amount of bile acids in your gallbladder.

A high-fiber diet could also help reduce your risk of gallstones by helping to control your weight. Being overweight is a well-known risk factor for gallbladder disease.

Caffeine. If you can't get moving until you've had your second cup of coffee in the morning, you might be protecting yourself from gallstones. A recent study found that men who drank two to three cups of coffee every day were 40 percent less likely to develop painful stones than those who didn't drink coffee.

Results of a later study found that coffee did not protect against gallstones, yet it did reduce symptoms in women who already had them. Researchers think the caffeine in coffee might prevent symptoms of gallstones, but not the gallstones themselves.

Vitamin C. Women are the unlucky recipients of more than two-thirds of all gallstones. You may be able to change your luck if you eat foods high in vitamin C, like citrus fruits, sweet red peppers, green peppers, strawberries, and cantaloupe.

In a large study, researchers found that a high blood level of vitamin C was associated with a lower rate of gallbladder disease in women, but not in men.

Scientists think women may be more likely to develop gallstones because estrogen increases the amount of cholesterol in the bile. Since most gallstones are made of excess cholesterol, vitamin C might be able to protect women because it helps convert cholesterol into bile acids.

Quick weight loss — a quick way to gallstones

Taking off extra weight is never easy. But doctors are now saying it can actually be downright painful, especially if you're a yo-yo dieter. That's because a new study shows that people who continually take off weight and put it back on are up to 70 percent more likely to get gallstones.

Being overweight is one of the main causes of gallstones, so taking off extra weight helps cut your risk. But it's important to lose the weight slowly and in such a way that you'll be able to keep it off. Otherwise, as the study shows, the weight loss does more harm than good.

The study followed 47,000 women for 16 years, recording their weight changes and gallstone problems. Moderate yo-yo dieters, women who went through cycles of losing 10 or more pounds only to gain them back quickly, had a 31-percent greater chance of getting gallstones than those who kept their weight steady. For severe yo-yo dieters, that number shot up to 68 percent.

Women, especially those between ages 20 and 60, have about twice the risk of men in developing gallstones. Pregnancy, birth control pills, and hormone replacement therapy raise your risk even more. Certain ethnic groups, such as Native Americans and Mexican-Americans, are also at higher risk.

If you are at risk for developing gallstones, particularly if you're trying to lose weight, try these preventive measures to help stop them before they start.

Team up with water. Water works wonders against cholesterol by helping to dissolve it before it has a chance to cause problems. Be sure to drink six to eight cups of water every day.

Try high C. Some experts believe a lack of vitamin C makes you more likely to develop gallstones. If you eat plenty of high-C foods, like citrus fruits, strawberries, and sweet red peppers, you might protect yourself from gallbladder attacks.

Don't skip meals. Going for long periods without eating decreases gallbladder contractions. If the gallbladder doesn't contract often enough, it's more likely to form gallstones.

Avoid ultra-low-calorie diets. If you eat too little fat, the gallbladder won't have any reason to contract and empty its bile. You need to eat a meal or snack of about 10 grams of fat for the gallbladder to contract normally.

Just remember, keeping your weight at a healthy level to begin with is the best way to avoid gallstones. But if those excess pounds sneak up on you, try to lose them slowly and sensibly. If you want to begin a strict weight loss program, discuss it with your doctor. He may decide you will benefit from ursodiol, a medication that can help prevent gallstones.

Surprising gallstone remedy

Are you willing to try an unusual home remedy for your gallstones? A chemical engineer wrote into the medical journal *The Lancet* with a self-treatment that he claimed worked on his wife's gallstones.

She drank one liter of apple juice every day for a week. On the seventh night, she drank a cup of olive oil just before bedtime, then slept on her left side all night. The next morning, she passed her gallstones.

While there is no scientific evidence to support this treatment, it is a fairly safe, gentle option. Just be sure to talk with your doctor before trying it.

Gout

Oust pain and inflammation naturally

"The gout," Charles Dickens once wrote, "is a complaint as arises from too much ease and comfort." Since ancient times, people believed gout only troubled kings, barons, and other rich folk who splurged on food and alcohol. That's why they called it "the disease of kings."

Experts now know gout is a form of arthritis that tends to run in families. If you suffer from gout, your body has problems dealing with uric acid, a natural by-product of metabolism. Either your body produces too much, or your kidneys can't flush it out. This causes uric acid to build up in your blood, leading to sudden and repeated attacks of gout.

In fact, you may fall asleep one night feeling fine, only to wake up with a red, aching, swollen big toe. That's how gout strikes. Crystals of uric acid are deposited in your joints, especially joints farthest from your chest, like your big toe, triggering the fiery inflammation. A painful attack can keep you bedridden for weeks.

Older people should be wary of taking aspirin frequently. As little as 75 milligrams (a little less than one children's aspirin) a day can affect the way your kidneys release uric acid.

If you have symptoms of gout, see your doctor. He can get at the root of the problem and prescribe medication to prevent future outbreaks. Failure to treat gout could cause permanently disfigured joints and kidney stones.

Being overweight and having high blood pressure are two major causes of gout. So play it safe – cut down on fatty foods; boost your daily intake of fruits, vegetables, and whole grains; and exercise regularly. Alcohol can also bring on an attack, making moderation a sensible practice if you drink at all.

Try adding some of these natural pain fighters to your menu to help relieve your gout.

Cherries. According to research from Michigan State University, if gout attacks, chew on some cherries. Dr. Muralee Nair, lead author of the study, suggests eating about 20 or so cherries a day to reduce the swelling and ache of a sudden gout attack. "Daily consumption of cherries," Nair says, "has the potential to reduce pain related to inflammation, arthritis, and gout."

Some researchers think cherries might work as well as drugs, without the side effects. Nair's test-tube studies show that cherry compounds are very effective when compared with aspirin, ibuprofen, and other nonsteroidal anti-inflammatory drugs (NSAIDs). These amazing cherry compounds are the same ones that give the fruit its red color. Called anthocyanins, they stop your body from producing prostaglandins, chemicals that cause inflammation. If eating a whole bowl of cherries sounds like a task fit for Hercules, dried cherries can provide a more concentrated dose.

Ginger and turmeric. According to the Arthritis Foundation, ginger and turmeric might be two more natural weapons against gout. Both spices contain curcumin, a phytochemical renown for its antioxidant and anti-inflammatory powers. It might even work as well as ibuprofen and other NSAIDs, according to recent research.

To try curcumin's healing powers, add fresh ginger to your next stir-fry or brew some ginger tea. And getting turmeric is as easy as ordering curry at your local Indian restaurant. If you have gallbladder disease or take NSAIDs or blood thinning medication, talk with your doctor before treating your gout with these spices.

Water. Your body needs at least eight 6-ounce glasses of water every day. Water not only helps prevent dehydration, it flushes out uric acid. Try to stick with plain old water. Sugary drinks, even the fashionable sports beverages that promise quick hydration, are loaded with empty calories.

Dairy. If you don't want another gout attack, soothe your system with dairy foods. According to a recent study from Canada, eating at least 30 grams of dairy protein a day can help keep the amount of uric acid circulating in your blood under control. Considering that one serving of yogurt has 12 grams of protein and a cup of milk has 8 grams, getting enough protein from dairy foods is easy to do.

Beware of purines

If you have gout, don't eat foods high in purines. They can make your gout worse. Purines cause your body to produce too much uric acid. This can trigger uric acid crystals to form in your joints, leading to inflammation and pain.

High purine foods include turkey, dried peas and beans, salmon, bacon, anchovies, liver, and cauliflower. Check with your doctor about following a low-purine diet.

Headaches

Head off pain with natural healers

Thank goodness headache remedies aren't what they used to be. In ancient times, people believed evil spirits caused this sometimes unbearable pain. They would drill holes in the sufferer's head to let these evil spirits out. The headache must have felt downright pleasant compared to the cure. Fortunately, today, many health experts believe you can find relief from headache pain just by watching what you eat.

About 90 percent of all headaches are tension headaches. These feel like you've got a tight band around your head causing pain in your forehead and temples or in the back of your head and neck. Less common are cluster headaches, with their typical sharp, sudden pain behind one eye.

Men get these much more often than women do. Yet, women have nearly three times as many migraine headaches as men. With a migraine, you feel a strong pain, usually on one side of your head. Light and sound bother your eyes and ears, and you might feel dizzy and sick to your stomach.

Many things can cause a headache – stress, fatigue, loud noise, bright lights, and changes in a woman's estrogen levels, such as during her period. Even skipping meals or eating the wrong foods, especially those containing substances that affect blood flow to your brain, can spell trouble. Some of the most common migraine triggers include red wine, cheese, and chocolate. Hot dogs, bacon, the Chinese food additive MSG, nuts, and citrus fruits could also lead to head pain.

The good news is you don't have to eliminate all of these foods from your diet. Different foods affect people differently. To find out if any foods give you trouble, try keeping a headache and food diary. If you see a pattern, like your headaches always come after you've snacked on a chocolate bar, you might think twice before eating that food.

Just as some foods can trigger headaches, some foods can help prevent them. To stop the pain before it starts, choose foods with plenty of these nutrients.

Magnesium. People who suffer with migraines, an estimated 28 million in the United States alone, have less of this mineral in their red blood cells and brain than other people. Because of this, researchers think a magnesium deficiency could cause migraines.

German researchers tested this idea and found that magnesium supplements helped reduce the number and severity of migraines. You would have to eat nearly 11 cups of oatmeal or 26 sweet potatoes to get as much natural magnesium as they used in this study, but don't get discouraged. Simply adding magnesium-rich foods, like brown rice, popcorn, broccoli, green peas, potatoes, shrimp, clams, and skim milk, to your daily meal plan could be enough to soothe your aching head.

Riboflavin. This B vitamin can be just as effective as aspirin in easing migraine pain. In one study, migraine sufferers who took daily supplements of riboflavin experienced as much improvement as those who took riboflavin plus aspirin. Like magnesium, this vitamin was studied in large doses. But that doesn't mean you can't boost your levels of riboflavin through diet. Milk, eggs, meat, poultry, fish, and green, leafy vegetables give you hefty amounts of this key vitamin.

Calcium and vitamin D. If you're a woman who gets migraines around the time of your period, extra calcium and vitamin D could mean fewer headaches and fewer PMS symptoms, too. This combination helped postmenopausal women with migraines as well. To get this therapy in one gulp, drink more vitamin D-fortified low-fat or fat-free milk.

Omega-3 fatty acids. Battles take place every day between omega-3 and omega-6 fatty acids – and your body is the battlefield. You need both of these essential fatty acids, and you must get them through your diet because your body can't make them on its own. On top of that, you need them in the right amounts.

When one type of fatty acid drastically outnumbers the other, things can go haywire. Experts say most people get more than enough omega-6 from a diet loaded with common vegetable oils. Too much of this omega-6 leads to too much signaling in your brain. This chaos triggers inflammation, which can give you all sorts of problems, including headaches.

"It's the fast-moving omega-6s that, when they're excessive, are the headache – literally and figuratively," says Dr. William Lands of the National Institutes of Health. "Billions of dollars are being spent to develop things that will slow down excessive omega-6 signaling." A cheaper strategy, and one you can control, is to get more omega-3 fatty acids that calm down the hyperactive omega-6. The best source of omega-3 is fish, especially fatty fish like salmon, mackerel, and tuna. But you'll also find it in walnuts, wheat germ, and some green, leafy vegetables.

Ginger. This spice has long been hailed for its powers to ward off nausea. Many herbal experts think eating ginger might help lessen the agony of a migraine attack, as well as the nausea that often comes with it.

Researchers from Denmark's Odense University gave a woman between 500 and 600 milligrams of powdered ginger at the first sign of a migraine. Within half an hour, she felt better. She then began taking 2 grams of powdered ginger every four hours. Eventually, she switched to eating fresh ginger every day. She reported having both fewer and less-intense migraines.

Although more research is needed to confirm ginger's effect on migraines, this information could help researchers solve the mystery of these excruciating headaches.

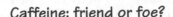

Caffeine: friend or foe?

In Operation Headache, caffeine acts as a double agent. On one hand, drinking too much caffeine or withdrawing from caffeine can trigger headaches. On the other, small amounts can help relieve the pain of a headache once it starts.

Caffeine constricts, or narrows, your blood vessels. This helps relieve pain because your blood vessels often swell before a headache. Caffeine also helps other headache medications work better, so you need less of them.

Just remember, caffeine is a drug – one you can grow to depend on. The National Headache Foundation recommends limiting yourself to two caffeinated beverages a day. If you drink a lot more coffee than that, cut back gradually. Giving it up all at once could trigger what's called a "rebound" headache.

7 clever natural remedies

Popping pills every time you get a headache can be a headache in itself. The next time your head throbs, try one of these natural cures. These folk remedies are trusty fixes for stress headaches.

Double-team the pain. While soaking in a steamy bath, hold an ice pack on your head. The combination of hot and cold relieves your headache by drawing blood away from your head and narrowing the blood vessels in your scalp.

Wrap it up. Try tying a bandana or handkerchief around your head, just above your brow. This could also reduce the blood flow in your scalp and get rid of the pounding in your head.

Treat your feet. With just one teaspoon of powdered mustard or ginger, you can turn a plastic basin of hot water into a fast headache cure. Just mix the powder into water that's as hot as you can stand. Then pull up your favorite chair, sit back, and let your feet soak for 15 minutes. It's important to cover the basin with a heavy towel to keep the heat in. Keep your eyes closed and your muscles relaxed for the full effect. Your headache should vanish by the time the water cools.

Serve up relief. To win match point against your headache, put two tennis balls in the toe of a tube sock and tie it tightly so the balls don't move. Then lie on your back and wedge the balls behind your neck, one on each side. They will relax your neck muscles, easing away headache-causing tension.

Try do-it-yourself massage. Sit in your favorite chair with your eyes closed. Begin massaging your temples and forehead, then work your way down to your neck and shoulders. Breathe slowly and deeply, and focus on relaxing your entire body.

Draw out the pain. To make a handy hot compress, heat some salt in a dry pan until it's warm but not too hot. Pour the salt into a thin dish towel and bundle it up. For pain in the front of your head, hold the compress to the back of your head and rub. The dry heat from the salt should relieve the ache.

Stop your headache cold. For a frozen compress, hold on to your old socks. Wet them and seal them in a zip-lock bag in your freezer. Use the whole sock if you want, or cut off the bottom and use the top.

Expert help for cluster headaches

At 2:00 a.m., you're suddenly jerked awake by a fierce pain on one side of your head. Your eyes may water, you may feel nauseated, your heart may beat wildly, and your blood pressure could shoot up. After about an hour, the agony goes away and you're able to sleep. But 10 minutes later, the sharp, burning pain returns. You've just experienced a cluster headache.

These headaches get their name from the fact that they come in bunches or "clusters." If you get one, you're likely to suffer from others within days, if not hours. They don't last long, but they do come back. Some sufferers can go for months or years without an attack, but when the clusters return, it may be for as long as two weeks of on-again, off-again torture.

The pain, which most people rate as worse than migraine pain, is sharp, stabbing, and severe. It usually affects one side of your head, but it can spread to your eyes, face, neck, and sometimes your whole head and entire upper body.

Understand the cause. Which came first, the chicken or the egg? Neurologists are asking a similar question – do cluster headaches cause brain abnormalities or do the abnormalities cause cluster headaches? Scientists at the Institute of Neurology in London studied people suffering from cluster headaches and, using state-of-the-art technology, found permanent flaws or defects in a specific section of their brain called the hypothalamus.

This area controls hunger, sex drive, and your body's natural 24-hour rhythm. Interestingly enough, this brain area shows unusual activity during a cluster headache.

This new information changes the way experts think about severe headaches, like cluster and migraine. Originally, neurologists believed your brain was healthy, but something odd happened to cause the headaches. Now, they think the brain itself could be flawed. This information could be the first step on the road to an effective treatment.

Avoid an attack. Although no one knows exactly what causes them, cluster headaches strike about six times more men than women. While you can't do anything about your gender, you can make some lifestyle changes that might help.

■ Stop smoking and limit alcohol. Heavy smokers or drinkers are more likely to suffer from cluster headaches – just another reason to cut these habits out of your life.

■ Get on a regular sleep cycle. This helps your body settle more easily into deep sleep patterns.

■ Avoid becoming overheated. A higher-than-normal body temperature may be one trigger that sets off a cluster headache. Sleeping in a cool bedroom may eliminate many cluster headache attacks.

Relieve the pain. Although experts don't have a sure-fire solution for cluster headaches, there are some things you can do to reduce how much they impact your life.

■ Put an ice pack or cold compress against your head to lessen the pain. As with other headaches, a heating pad may work better for you – experiment to find out.

■ Try holding your hands in ice water until it becomes uncomfortable. It's an odd remedy, but some people say it works.

Even if you find ways to lessen the pain of a cluster attack, see your doctor for a checkup. You'll want to rule out any other problems. Also, she might be able to prescribe medication to help manage your pain.

Hearing loss

Super strategies to improve your hearing

Your ears are not like other parts of your body. Working them harder won't make them stronger. The delicate mechanisms that make up your inner ear are very sensitive. You can damage your hearing gradually doing ordinary, everyday activities without knowing you're doing any harm.

While you can't isolate yourself completely from harsh noises, there are steps you can take to minimize your exposure – and there are ways to cope with hearing loss.

Quiet your world. The more noise you cut from your day, the better it is for your ears. Try reducing noise from appliances, printers, and typewriters by placing them on rubber mats. Block out street and other outside noise with drapes, fabric wall hangings, and double-paned windows. The best absorber of indoor noise is a plush carpet.

Insulate your ears. If you're going to be working at a loud task, prepare beforehand. Using power tools, riding motorcycles or snowmobiles, and discharging firearms are all common activities loud enough to cause serious damage to your ears over time. To prevent this, wear foam earplugs. They are inexpensive, and you can buy them at hardware or discount stores.

Stop abusing noise. A lot of people use noise to cover noise, which only makes things harder on your delicate ears. If a loud noise is bothering you, don't turn up the TV or stereo to drown it out. Instead, see if there's any way to stifle the noise.

Get used to quiet. Try lowering the volume on your radio, TV, and headset. People often listen at a certain volume more out of habit than necessity. If someone standing nearby can hear sounds coming from your headphones, you've got them turned up too loud. Try keeping the noise in your home to a bare minimum.

Give them rest. Your ears need time to recover, especially after a really loud day. Giving them a few hours of low-noise time can help them recuperate.

Don't strain. Extreme physical stress can raise the level of pressure in your ears to a dangerous level and cause damage to your hearing. Use extra caution when lifting heavy objects or exerting yourself in any way.

Exercise regularly. Add hearing to the list of things exercise helps. Exercise improves the circulation of blood to your inner ear where it helps keep hearing mechanisms, such as your sound-detecting hair cells, in good working order.

Ditch the wax. If you think your hearing is going, check your earwax. Cleaning out your ears might clear up your hearing.

Check your medicine. Some drugs can cause or contribute to hearing loss. Aspirin, furosemide, neomycin, and gentamicin are common culprits. If you take any of these drugs, have your hearing checked regularly.

Talk in corners. Standing in a corner puts two surfaces behind you to reflect sound and make it easier to hear. It creates the same effect as cupping your hand over your ear — it helps to catch the sound and direct it where it's needed.

Speak up. If you are having trouble hearing someone, ask them to speak in a deeper tone of voice. When hearing damage occurs, high-pitched noises are among the first you lose. Lower tones are easier to pick up.

Wear a hearing aid. Hearing aids can work wonders for you, and they are getting better and more affordable every day. Be sure to have yours fitted by a doctor. Although dealers know their product, only a doctor can examine you, find out the cause of your hearing loss, and suggest alternative treatments.

Tune in to the latest technology. If your hearing loss is permanent, but not total, there are many things you can do around the house to make it easier to hear. Some of the latest helpers available are amplifiers for your phone, TV, and VCR. Just about anything that makes noise can be retooled to make the noise louder.

Protect yourself at home. For safety's sake, make sure every alarm in your home is loud enough to alert you. Test the buzzer on your doorbell, your oven, security system, smoke detectors, and the ring of your telephone. If you can't hear these sounds, they can be replaced or supplemented with flashing lights. Closed captioning, which allows you to read along with what's being said on screen, is available on most new televisions. The technology of TDD (Telecommunication Device for the Deaf) helps make phone calls easier. More and more companies and agencies are getting TDD lines to accommodate the needs of the hearing impaired.

Get tested for free. For a quick, free test of your hearing, call Dial-a-Hearing Test at 1-800-222-EARS (3277). They'll give you a local number you can call to take a two-minute hearing test over the phone.

Learn the facts. To learn more about what options and opportunities are available to people with hearing problems, contact one of the organizations listed here.

National Association of the Deaf
Phone: (301) 587-1788
TDD: (301) 587-1789

American Speech-Language-Hearing Association
Phone: (800) 638-8255
TDD: Same

Alexander Graham Bell Association for the Deaf

Phone: (202) 337-5220

TDD: (202) 337-5221

Now hear this: Vacuuming can harm ears

Explosions and machine gun fire can put a soldier's hearing, as well as his life, at risk. But you don't have to be a veteran of the battlefield to suffer noise-induced hearing loss. Many objects in your own home can also damage your ears – vacuum cleaners, garbage disposals, leaf blowers, and shop tools.

Sound is measured in units called decibels. To get an idea of how loud a decibel is, normal conversation is about 60 decibels. Any sound above 75 decibels has the potential to cause hearing loss. A sudden loud noise, like an explosion, or loud noises over a long period of time, like continuous sounds in your workplace, can damage the delicate hair cells or hearing nerves in your ears. This can lead to hearing loss or tinnitus.

According to the American Tinnitus Association, everyday noises that might cause hearing loss include:

- Blow dryer – 100 decibels

- Subway – 100 decibels

- Power lawn mower – 105 decibels

- Chainsaw – 105 decibels

- Motorcycle – 120 decibels

- Fireworks – 120 decibels

- Shotgun blast – 140 decibels

Recreational activities like woodworking, riding snowmobiles or go-carts, target shooting, and hunting also endanger your ears. In fact, a recent University of Wisconsin study found that men who regularly engage in target shooting are 57 percent more likely to have hearing loss than those who don't.

And the more years you hunt, the greater your risk of hearing loss. Unfortunately, a third of the target shooters and almost all of the hunters reported never wearing hearing protection.

Even if you don't use firearms, noise can mean big trouble for your ears. More than 30 million people are exposed to high-decibel sounds on a regular basis, whether at work, at play, or at home. Here's how to protect yourself.

Know your enemy. Be aware of what noises might harm your ears. Make sure your family, friends, co-workers, and children are protected against noises louder than 75 decibels.

Block your ears. Wear earplugs or earmuffs when you participate in a loud activity. These can prevent both kinds of hearing loss – that caused by a brief impulse (explosion) or the kind caused by continuous exposure. You can find them at hardware or sporting goods stores.

Get a check-up. Sometimes hearing loss is so gradual you might not notice it until it's too late. Schedule an examination by an ear, nose, and throat specialist and a hearing test by an audiologist, a health professional who can detect and measure hearing loss.

Taking these precautions will make your day-to-day encounters with noise a little easier on your ears. And remember, before you plug in that vacuum cleaner, put in some earplugs.

Safest ways to clean your ears

If you're like most people, earwax is something you never think about, but maybe you should. This yellowish secretion protects your inner ear from potentially damaging things, like sand, dirt, and insects.

Too much earwax can make hearing difficult. In extreme cases, it can block the ear canal. Having very hairy or narrow ears can make the problem even worse.

If you are having trouble with earwax, follow this top-notch advice from the experts.

Toss aside the cotton swabs. Did your mother ever tell you not to stick anything smaller than your elbow in your ear? She was right. Trying to pick at earwax with your fingers, tweezers, or other sharp objects could cause serious injury. Even cotton swabs are a no-no. Doctors say a swab is more likely to push the wax deeper into your ear.

Flush it away. Fill a bowl or bathroom sink with warm water. Using a rubber ball syringe, turn your head to one side and flush one ear at a time with water, dropping the water in gently. Never apply more than just the slightest bit of pressure. Remember, you're trying to soften the wax, not blast it out.

Try a drop of oil. If warm water hasn't done the trick, try a different approach. Use an eyedropper to place a couple of drops of oil – baby, vegetable, or mineral – into your ear. Hold it in with a cotton ball for a few minutes, then wipe away the excess. Over a day or two, the oil should start to break up the wax. You can also use this technique with hydrogen peroxide, glycerin, or a warm water and vinegar solution.

Chomp down on buildup. Your body's natural defense against earwax buildup isn't an active pinkie finger – it's chewing. The chewing motion of your teeth and jaw actually breaks up earwax and keeps your ear canal in good working order. People who don't chew their food very well often have trouble with earwax.

Cut back on fat. Research has shown that saturated fat, found mostly in foods of animal origin, causes your ears to produce too much earwax. So take it easy on your hearing while you take it easy on your heart – cut back on saturated fat.

Heartburn

Foods that help put out the fire

More than 60 million Americans suffer from heartburn and indigestion. If you burp a lot, sometimes with a burning taste in your mouth, and feel bloated and uncomfortable after meals, you're probably one of them. These symptoms often get worse during times of stress. Maybe you have resigned yourself to the discomfort, figuring nothing will help the burning feeling in your gut. But don't ignore it. Even though heartburn is not a disease, it could be a symptom of something more serious.

That burning in your throat after eating is probably acid reflux. It happens when stomach acid washes back up your throat. This can lead to nausea and vomiting. Acid reflux, also called GERD (gastroesophageal reflux disease) is serious because it can damage your esophagus and lead to severe bleeding.

It also increases your risk of esophageal cancer. If your indigestion makes you vomit blood or comes with a severe, burning pain in your stomach, see your doctor immediately. You might have gastritis, an inflammation of the stomach.

What you eat and the medicines you take affect your digestive system. For instance, eating too much fat and red meat and not enough fruits and vegetables can cause acid reflux. Taking antibiotics may wipe out both good and bad bacteria, leading to indigestion and diarrhea. And constantly popping antacids for heartburn can backfire by prompting your body to make more acid.

Why not get to the root of your heartburn – what you are or aren't eating. If your doctor has ruled out disease, try healing your heartburn and indigestion by making a few simple changes in your daily eating plan.

Water. Drink plenty of water during the day. Six 8-ounce glasses should help with your indigestion. Water washes acid out of your throat and dilutes the acid in your stomach. But don't drink liquids with meals since you need stomach acid to digest your food. An hour before or after is best.

Dr. Fereydoon Batmanghelidj, author of *Your Body's Many Cries For Water*, says your body needs lots of water for proper digestion. Unfortunately, if you fill up with coffee and colas, you lose water since the caffeine in these drinks signals your kidneys to pump water out of your body.

Dr. B., as his patients call him, has had much success treating indigestion with plain, old water. "Dyspeptic pain," he explains, "is the most important signal for the human body. It denotes dehydration. It is a thirst signal of the body. It can occur in the very young as well as in older people."

The next time your stomach cries for help, give it several glasses of water to quench the fire.

Yogurt. Yogurt is a "probiotic" food, which means it helps good bacteria grow. Even if most milk products cause your indigestion to kick in, you can probably eat yogurt since the friendly bacteria in yogurt have predigested the milk sugar for you.

Yogurt is especially good if you have recently taken antibiotics. To get these helpful bacteria, and not just milk and sugar, read the label and make sure the yogurt has active cultures. Buy plain yogurt and flavor it with some fresh blueberries, strawberries, raspberries, or peaches.

Fruits, veggies, and grains. Replace high-fat meats and fried foods that promote stomach acid with low-acid fruits, vegetables, and whole grains, like whole-wheat bread and brown rice. And the grains should help soak up excess acid. Stay away from acidic foods, like tomatoes, oranges, grapefruits, radishes, alcohol, coffee, tea, and cola.

Bitter plants. Dogs may be smarter than people when it comes to soothing an upset stomach. When a dog's stomach hurts, it finds some bitter grass to eat. That's pretty smart since bitter herbs help get your digestive juices flowing.

Some people have too much stomach acid, and some have too little, especially older people. If you don't have enough acid, your food may sit undigested in your stomach too long, causing pain. To fight this kind of indigestion, eat bitter plants like watercress, endive, dandelion, artichokes, and grated orange peel – but don't eat the orange.

Ginger, a bitter spice, has been used for centuries to treat indigestion. Steep a teaspoon of grated ginger in hot water for 10 minutes, and drink throughout the day as needed.

Chamomile tea. Another ancient remedy, chamomile tea settles the stomach and helps digestion. Drink a cup between meals three or four times a day. You can buy chamomile flower heads at a natural food store. Steep a heaping tablespoon 10 to 15 minutes before drinking. Be careful if you are allergic to ragweed. You might also be allergic to chamomile.

15 surprising ways to cool the heat

If heartburn pain is a frequent guest at your table, here are some things you can do to make your life more comfortable.

Eat less, more often. Small, frequent meals, say four to six light helpings a day, are healthier than three large ones. Avoid stuffing yourself and eating just before bedtime. Don't even lie down for four hours after eating.

Think bland. Fatty and spicy dishes will irritate your stomach lining and esophagus. Some of the worst offenders are tomato products, onions, and peppers. Acidic foods, like citrus juices, can also cause irritation.

Watch what you drink. You should cut down on coffee, tea, alcoholic beverages, and whole milk. These liquids tend to irritate your stomach lining.

Chew it to cool it. The more you chew, the more acid-neutralizing saliva you produce. Take small bites and chew your food slowly and thoroughly. After eating, chew a piece of sugarless gum. Sucking on sugarless hard candy during the day may also help, but avoid peppermint-flavored candy.

Timing is everything. Remember to drink liquids about an hour before or after meals to keep your stomach from bloating. Don't mix foods and liquids.

Improve your posture. Sit up straight when you're eating, never stand or lie down. And don't bend over immediately after eating. This forces food and digestive acids back up into your esophagus.

Avoid tight clothes. Don't wear clothes and belts that fit tightly around your stomach. When you're shopping, choose clothes that fit loosely at your waistline.

Slim down. If you are overweight, losing those extra pounds might help relieve your heartburn symptoms. The extra weight squeezes your stomach and forces the acidic digestive juices back up into your esophagus.

Do one thing at a time. Don't eat while you're working, playing, or driving.

Give up smoking. And if you're already trying to quit, don't wear your nicotine patch to bed. The nicotine the patch releases can cause heartburn.

Get support while you sleep. Use 4- to 6-inch wooden blocks or bricks to raise the head of your bed. Or put a foam wedge beneath your upper body. This keeps digestive juices flowing down instead of up as you sleep.

Turn to the left. A recent study found that sleeping on your left side could reduce your risk of heartburn. People in the study who slept on their backs had more episodes of heartburn than others. However, stomach acid took longer to clear out of the esophagus in those who slept on their right sides, allowing more time for the acid to damage the esophagus.

Down the hatch. Drink plenty of water with your medications, and don't lie down after swallowing a pill. This helps the pills go down and stay down. Drinking water throughout the day will also help keep digestive acids out of your esophagus.

Take it easy. Avoid straining and heavy lifting. This causes your abdominal muscles to contract and squeeze the contents of your stomach into your esophagus.

Know your medications. Talk with your doctor if you are taking any heart or blood pressure medicines. These can affect the sphincter between your esophagus and stomach, allowing acid to back up into your esophagus.

If your heartburn becomes severe and is accompanied by nausea, sweating, weakness, fainting, breathlessness, or pain that extends from your chest to your arm or jaw, you might have something much worse than a pepperoni pizza that didn't sit well. These are symptoms of a heart attack. Call for help.

Heart disease

Amazing foods that keep your heart healthy

Just as a traffic jam can bring a city to a standstill, gridlock in your blood vessels can do all sorts of damage to your body. If your blood has trouble moving through your arteries, you're at greater risk for a heart attack, stroke, varicose veins, and a host of other diseases. Fortunately, you can improve your circulation with the help of these delicious foods.

Grape juice. After years of taking grapes apart and examining the pieces, scientists have decided they are healthiest just as they are – whole. Grape seed extract and grape skin extract each, on its own, does little to stop your blood from clotting and blocking your arteries. But when the two substances are combined, the mixture can reduce platelet clumping by 91 percent. And that's why grape juice, made from whole grapes, is a heart-smart choice. Two glasses of purple grape juice a day can make a big difference.

Tea. If you have heart disease, you know you run a greater risk of having a stroke. But adding a simple and relaxing habit might change the numbers in your favor. New research shows that drinking black tea can help open up your blood vessels, which might have narrowed because of heart disease.

When study participants drank four cups of tea daily for four weeks, their blood vessels expanded to near normal size. The changes took place within just a few hours of drinking the first cup of tea.

Researchers knew caffeine wasn't responsible for the change because people given a caffeine pill didn't have the same results. They thought flavonoids – strong antioxidants found in tea – were likely at work. More studies are needed, but in the meantime, why not try tea instead of coffee? Unlike a new drug with unknown side effects, tea has always been considered safe. In fact, people have been drinking black tea for centuries without any trouble.

Nuts and seeds. Because they are rich in both unsaturated fats and vitamin E, foods like walnuts, sesame seeds, and almonds provide a one-two punch against heart attack, stroke, and other serious circulation problems.

Unsaturated fats help prevent clots and lower cholesterol, which can clog your arteries and make it harder for your blood to get through. Vitamin E stops LDL, or bad, cholesterol from clinging to your artery walls, decreasing your risk for heart attack or stroke. In one study, women who took vitamin E supplements for more than two years had 41 percent fewer heart attacks.

Low levels of this antioxidant vitamin are also associated with diabetes, rheumatoid arthritis, and intermittent claudication. Other sources of unsaturated fats are fish and olive oil. You can find vitamin E in wheat germ, vegetable oils, and green leafy vegetables.

Fruits and vegetables. These nutritional powerhouses have a lot to offer, including fiber, vitamins, and minerals. Along with vitamin E, the antioxidants beta carotene (which your body turns into vitamin A) and vitamin C help lower your risk for stroke. Vitamin C strengthens your small blood vessels and thins your blood so it flows more smoothly, while vitamin A rejuvenates your tissues and cell linings. Both also boost your immune system and rid your body of toxins.

Eat carrots, plums, tomatoes, and watercress for a healthy dose of these important nutrients. But don't stop there. Asparagus, cantaloupe, pinto beans, beets, and leafy greens provide folic acid, a B vitamin that protects your heart. Many grain products in the United States are now fortified with folic acid because experts estimated that 50,000 fewer Americans would die from heart attacks each year if manufacturers added folic acid to breads, cereals, and other products.

Fish. If you want to keep your heart healthy, eat fish more often. A large study on male doctors found that those who ate at least one fish meal a week were 52 percent less likely to die from a sudden heart attack than those who ate fish less than once a month.

Omega-3 fatty acids are the heart heroes in fish. Research indicates that omega-3 can lower your blood pressure, reduce the stickiness of your blood, and help regulate your heartbeat. Fatty fish, such as tuna and salmon, contain lots of omega-3. If you're not a big fan of fish, you can also get omega-3 in some green leafy vegetables, like spinach and kale.

Flaxseed. Flaxseed oil and flaxseed give you a good amount of alpha-linolenic acid, a type of omega-3 fatty acid that lowers blood pressure and your risk for stroke. This wonder food, once praised by Gandhi, also fights arthritis, heart disease, diabetes, stomach disorders, and even mental problems. It also protects against cancers of the breast, prostate, and colon.

Use flaxseed oil in salad dressings, soups, or sauces, and sprinkle flaxseed on cereals and salads. Bake with flaxseed flour, or stir in some flaxseed for crunchy cookies, breads, or muffins. But add flaxseed to your diet slowly – too much, too fast can give you gas if you're not used to it. You'll also find alpha-linolenic acid in walnuts, as well as walnut or canola oil.

Beans. By providing plenty of protein without artery-clogging cholesterol and saturated fat, beans, like pinto beans, and other legumes make wonderful alternatives to meat. If you switch just half of your protein intake from meat to legume sources, you could lower your cholesterol by 10 percent or more.

Beans are also high in fiber, which can protect your heart and shrink your stroke risk, and have been shown to lower cholesterol. And when your protein occasionally comes from beans and other vegetables instead of meat, you improve your chances of avoiding cancer and liver damage.

Discover the secret of a funny fruit

Ounce for ounce, what fruit contains the most vitamin C? If you said an orange, you'd be wrong. That honor belongs to a fuzzy little fruit you should eat more often – the kiwifruit.

When comparing kiwis and oranges, the kiwi comes out ahead more than 2 to 1. One orange contains about 45 milligrams (mg) of vitamin C, but one kiwifruit contains about 98 mg of vitamin C. The kiwi is also loaded with potassium, another key nutrient in the battle against heart disease and stroke.

Get protection from garlic

Picture a rubber band that's been sitting in a drawer for a few years. It's no longer soft and stretchy but has turned hard and cracks easily. Now picture your arteries. They begin life just like that rubber band, soft and stretchy. But as you get older, they become stiff and inflexible – simply a natural part of aging.

Only now this stiffness means every time your heart beats, your arteries don't spring back as easily as they used to, and you can end up with high blood pressure. Blood doesn't flow as smoothly through these stiffened arteries either, which causes a buildup of fats, leading to atherosclerosis. That means a greater chance of a heart attack or stroke.

Here's where garlic comes in. This small, unassuming herb, which has been used in cooking and healing for thousands of years, can put that spring back into your arteries – and your life. Researchers in Germany found that garlic pills kept the main artery to the heart soft and flexible. In fact, the older the test volunteers were, the greater the benefit.

Although researchers are still studying exactly how garlic works this minor miracle, they do know it helps improve blood flow in your arteries, keeping them, and your heart, strong and healthy.

But garlic doesn't stop there. It contributes to your health in several other ways.

Blasts away blood clots. Research has proven that garlic makes your blood less sticky, less likely to clot. Fewer clots mean less chance of heart attack and stroke.

But to get this heart-saving advantage, you need to take low doses over a long period of time. An occasional high dose just doesn't do the trick. Make garlic an everyday part of your cooking style and stop blood clots before they start.

Shields your arteries. If you've read anything at all about antioxidants, you know flavonoids provide powerful protection against artery damage. Nutritionists were thrilled to discover these natural disease-fighting compounds in many fruits and vegetables, as well as garlic.

Conquers cholesterol. Several recent studies claim there is no hard evidence that garlic lowers cholesterol. There are, however, dozens of past studies declaring just the opposite, that garlic prevents the build up of fat and cholesterol in your arteries, reduces triglycerides, and increases HDL cholesterol. In one of those studies, eating a fresh clove of garlic every day for 16 weeks reduced cholesterol by an amazing 20 percent.

Since garlic has been proven healthy in so many other ways, you can't go wrong adding it to your menu. In fact, if cholesterol is a concern for you, plan two or three meals a week around garlic and fatty fish, like salmon. This combination seems to lower cholesterol better than either one alone.

Boycotts high blood pressure. Garlic is best known for loosening up those arteries and allowing your blood to flow more easily. This means less stress on your heart and better circulation. Some studies suggest garlic can lower blood pressure by several points.

All these studies tested various forms of garlic, including garlic powder, garlic extract, and garlic oil, as well as garlic cloves. Although experts aren't saying if you get more benefit from fresh garlic over garlic supplements, most nutritionists agree it's a good idea to use whole foods whenever possible.

Supplements can be missing vital, health-saving benefits found only in a whole food. If you are trying to figure out equal amounts, one clove of garlic is about the same as 1,000 milligrams (mg) of a garlic supplement.

2 herbs that improve heart health

Using plants for medicine is nothing new. In fact, many modern medicines were originally created from plants. Digitalis, long used in the treatment of heart failure, first came from the dried leaf of the foxglove plant.

Even though herbs can provide natural and inexpensive health protection, talk with your doctor before taking any herbs. Some herbs can interact with medication.

Ginkgo biloba. Aspirin can make your blood less sticky, which can protects you from a heart attack or stroke. Unfortunately, aspirin can upset your stomach and sometimes cause internal bleeding. But now you have another option. A supplement called ginkgo biloba, made from a tree that existed in China before the ice age, can also do the job.

Laboratory studies show that ginkgo keeps blood clots from forming, making it a good stroke fighter. Although it works much like aspirin, side effects are rare.

Ginkgo can also relieve symptoms of intermittent claudication, a condition that causes severe pain in your calf muscles when you walk because of poor circulation.

Many people find they can walk further without pain when they take this supplement. In addition, there are usually few side effects. Herbal experts recommend taking 120 to 160 milligrams (mg) a day with meals for relief.

Horse chestnut. Several studies show this seed extract helps people with varicose veins and chronic venous insufficiency, a condition where the valves in your veins don't work properly. Blood has trouble making its way back to your heart so it builds up in your lower legs.

Taking horse chestnut seed extract for two weeks can reduce swelling in your calves and ankles, as well as relieve leg pain, itching, and fatigue. Make sure your extract has 100 to 150 mg of escin, the active ingredient in this herb.

7 simple steps to spotless arteries

You've heard the expression "Cleanliness is next to godliness." That goes for your arteries as well. With the right diet, you can scrub clogged arteries clean. Just follow these guidelines from the U.S. Department of Agriculture and the U.S. Department of Health and Human Services.

Eat a variety of foods. In order to get the right balance of nutrients, eat foods from all food groups. They each offer something unique and necessary to good health.

Maintain a healthy weight. A major risk factor for heart disease is excess weight. A good eating plan of low-fat, whole-grain foods will keep the pounds off and your heart healthy.

Trim the fat. Keep your total fat, saturated fat, and cholesterol intakes low.

Load up on plant foods. By eating plenty of vegetables, fruits, and grain products, you'll be giving your body a natural source of vitamins, minerals, and antioxidants.

Watch the sweets. Use table sugar and sugared products in moderation. Learn to snack on fruit instead.

Lower your salt. Whether it comes out of a shaker or shows up in processed foods, salt should be a small part of your diet.

Limit the alcohol. Drink only in moderation. Consuming one or two drinks a day is usually considered moderate drinking.

There are lots of small, easy changes you can make in your daily eating habits that will mean big heart benefits. Be patient and don't give up. It could take your body several months to adjust to these changes in diet.

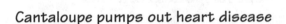

Cantaloupe pumps out heart disease

There's safety in numbers. Especially when you're facing a number of dangers. High blood pressure, cholesterol, and homocysteine all contribute to heart disease. Fortunately, mouthwatering cantaloupe has enough weapons to counter all of these threats.

◆ Potassium. This mineral keeps your blood pressure under wraps, particularly when you watch your sodium intake. And cantaloupe contains plenty of potassium.

◆ Vitamin C. That same cup of cubed cantaloupe gives you more than 100 percent of the RDA for vitamin C. That's good because according to researchers from the Boston University School of Medicine, vitamin C works to lower blood pressure and may improve blood flow in people with chronic heart failure.

◆ Folate. This member of the B-vitamin family can control homocysteine, a substance that's known to trigger strokes and heart attacks.

◆ Fiber. Cantaloupe contains soluble fiber, which can dramatically lower your cholesterol. One cantaloupe gives you 5 grams of fiber.

Exercise — the most powerful healer on earth

Health experts say a lack of exercise is as much a heart disease risk factor as high cholesterol, cigarette smoking, and high blood pressure. Here's how exercising can help you strengthen your heart.

Peels off pounds. Carrying around excess weight is a sure route to high cholesterol, high blood pressure, and diabetes. If you want to lose weight, you must burn up more calories than you take in, and exercise can help. The best results come from combining aerobic exercise, like brisk walking or jogging, with a low-fat diet.

Keeps arteries flexible. As you age, your blood vessels become less flexible. When your muscles signal a need for more oxygen and nutrients, your arteries can't dilate to allow more blood to flow through. Your heart has to work harder, which increases your heart rate and blood pressure. By exercising regularly, you are actually keeping your arteries in shape, not just your muscles.

Improves cholesterol levels. Regular exercise lowers total and bad LDL cholesterol and increases good HDL cholesterol. Some studies have found that exercise can improve cholesterol levels as much as medication, without the side effects.

Lowers heart attack risk. Do you often worry that exercising will bring on a heart attack? If you never work out and suddenly do something strenuous, there is some risk. The good news is regular exercise will lower this risk. If your heart is used to moderate exercise, say four or five workouts a week, then some heavy exertion shouldn't be dangerous. Better pass that snow shovel on to someone else if you don't exercise regularly.

Speeds recovery time. If you have suffered a heart attack or other heart-related injury, here's good motivation to start some kind of exercise program. Studies have shown that if you become active right away, you are more likely to be discharged earlier from the hospital and return to your usual activities.

Lifts your spirits. When you do something physical, you feel better. Although depression is common after a heart attack, it will usually go away on its own. In the meantime, exercise will help to lessen that gloomy feeling. You'll feel an emotional lift knowing you're doing something good for your heart. You'll also feel a very real physical charge when your body releases chemicals called endorphins, which block pain and give you a sense of well-being.

Drug-free ways to triumph over heart disease

Heart disease is a killer, and the best way to avoid being a victim is to practice prevention. If you already have heart disease or high blood pressure, or even if you've had heart surgery, you still have the power to increase your odds of beating this disease. And the most powerful weapons you have might be your mind, your church, and your family.

Researchers studying people who had undergone angioplasty found that those who scored low on measures of self-esteem, optimism, and being in control of their lives were two-and-a-half times more likely to have a heart attack or require another angioplasty or bypass surgery.

Optimism. If you have heart problems, it could help you live longer. According to the latest research, a positive attitude can increase your chances of surviving heart problems. Studies find that people with a positive attitude, high self-esteem, and a sense of control over their lives do better after a heart attack.

A similar study followed people who had undergone heart bypass surgery for six months after the surgery. Researchers found that the most optimistic people were 50 percent less likely to be hospitalized again for subsequent heart problems, like infection, angina, or a second operation to reopen their clogged arteries.

And an optimistic attitude may help you live longer, even if you don't have heart problems. One 30-year study found that people who scored high on the pessimistic end of a personality test had a 19 percent greater risk of dying earlier than people who scored high on optimism.

Meditation. Your doctor can give you medicine to help lower your blood pressure, but about half of the people stop taking their medicine after one year, usually because of unpleasant side effects. Proper diet and exercise will also help lower blood pressure, but many people are not willing to follow that advice.

Another way to lower your blood pressure is to practice meditation. Meditation helps you relax, and it opens up your blood vessels, making it easier for your heart to pump blood throughout your body. Find an instructor who can teach you proper meditation techniques, and you might be able to lower your blood pressure without medication.

A study on African-Americans with high blood pressure showed that the participants who practiced meditation for three months reduced their systolic blood pressure (the top number) an average of 10 to 12 points and their diastolic blood pressure (the bottom number) six to eight points.

These reductions are similar to those achieved by taking blood pressure medication. But remember – follow your doctor's advice. Don't stop taking your medication without his approval.

Prayer. When you're in distress, saying a prayer can make you feel better, but that's not all. Researchers found incredible evidence that people who are prayed for benefit, even when they don't realize they're being prayed for.

In one study, the first names of heart patients were given to a group of people from various religions who prayed for them daily for four weeks. The patients never met the people who were praying for them, and they weren't even aware that anyone was praying for them. Nevertheless, researchers found an 11-percent reduction in scores of heart disease severity in the prayer group compared with a group that wasn't prayed for.

Family support. Numerous studies have found that strong social support can lower your risk of disease. People with heart disease may especially benefit from a supportive family.

A recent study found that married people with supportive relationships respond better to stress than couples with a low level of social support. Researchers studied 45 couples and measured their blood pressure and other responses to stress.

Men with supportive relationships showed a lower increase in blood pressure, as well as less constriction of their blood vessels. Women with supportive relationships had less constriction of blood vessels, but the increase in blood pressure was about the same. Researchers say these improvements in stress response translate into less stress on your heart.

Hemorrhoids

8 ways to find relief

Even though half of adults over age 50 have hemorrhoids, that doesn't mean you should ignore them. These swollen veins can occur inside the rectum or bulge outside the anus. Both kinds can become itchy and painful, and they can also bleed.

There's no reason to live with the pain. Give these natural remedies a try, but if your condition worsens or doesn't improve within seven days, or if bleeding occurs, see your doctor.

Fight back with fiber. The number one way to prevent and treat hemorrhoids is to add more fiber to your diet. Fiber will help you avoid constipation, soften your stool, and relieve the pressure on your hemorrhoids.

Try to get about 25 to 30 grams of fiber each day. Good sources are bran, whole grain foods, potatoes, beans, and fresh fruits. To really get things moving, eat more vegetables, like cabbage, corn, parsnips, brussels sprouts, cauliflower, peas, asparagus, and carrots.

Foods low in fiber will only slow up the process and make your stools harder to pass. Avoid ice cream, soft drinks, cheese, white bread, and meat. Some people find that certain foods, like coffee, nuts, or spicy foods, make their hemorrhoid symptoms worse.

Take it "sitting" down. If your hemorrhoids are inflamed, soaking in a few inches of warm water with your knees raised will really ease your pain. Try three 15-minute soaks a day to soothe your uncomfortable symptoms. Don't make the water too hot, and don't add anything like bubble bath or Epsom salts. These can irritate swollen veins. Relax in your bathtub or try Sitz Baths. You can find them at your local pharmacy very reasonably priced.

Practice proper bathroom etiquette. Straining during a bowel movement is one of the major causes of hemorrhoids. To prevent this, take a footstool into the bathroom and prop up your feet. If you don't have a stool, anything that raises your feet at least a few inches will do.

Try gently lubricating the area, inside and out, with nonpetroleum jelly first. You may find bowel movements less irritating.

And although you shouldn't rush the process, don't sit too long either. Enjoying your favorite magazine for more than a few minutes increases the pressure on the veins in your rectum. The longer you sit, the more your veins swell.

Last, but not least, clean the area well. If it's particularly sensitive after a bowel movement, wipe with a soft, moist tissue or baby wipes instead of regular toilet tissue.

Flush it out. Six to eight glasses of liquid each day will flush out your digestive system and keep it from becoming impacted. Stay away from alcohol because it draws water from your body and causes constipation.

Stay active. Hemorrhoids should not restrict your normal exercise routine. In fact, it's more important than ever for you to exercise every day – for two reasons.

First of all, moving around instead of sitting takes pressure off the veins in your rectum. And secondly, exercise helps prevent constipation, one of the main causes of hemorrhoids. Just avoid heavy lifting and any activity that causes you to strain.

Slim down. Being overweight is often a consequence of an inactive lifestyle and poor diet. Changing these two things will improve your health, including your hemorrhoids.

Cool the heat. If your hemorrhoids are painfully swollen, take this as an excuse to rest. Stay in bed for a few hours with an ice pack on your anal area.

Reach for over-the-counter help. There are several products you can buy for different kinds of hemorrhoid relief. Bulk stool softeners are helpful, but stay away from laxatives. Diarrhea is just as bad for hemorrhoids as constipation. External creams or ointments for pain, swelling, and itching usually contain a lubricant to relieve irritation, but nonpetroleum jelly does the same job. If you choose a commercial product, these are some helpful ingredients:

- Hydrocortisone – relieves inflammation and itching.

- Anesthetics (benzocaine, pramoxine) – can numb the pain.

- Vasoconstrictors (ephedrine, phenylephrine) – reduce swelling and relieve itching.

- Astringents (witch hazel, zinc oxide) – help shrink swollen blood vessels.

- Counterirritants (camphor) – soothe and comfort the area.

- Aloe vera gel – reduces irritation.

Particular brands may list other ingredients, such as wound-healing agents and antiseptics, but not all of these have been proven useful.

Hiccups

17 hiccup remedies that really work

Man can walk on the moon and create computers the size of a fingernail, but hiccups remain a mystery. Unfortunately, curing them is just as puzzling. Although doctors have tried everything from drugs to hypnosis, these old-fashioned home remedies seem to work just as well.

Change the pressure in your sinuses. By plugging up your ear canal, you are increasing the pressure inside your sinuses, forcing the muscle spasm that caused the hiccup to relax. Try one of these for relief.

- plug up one ear with your finger

- plug both ears and drink a glass of water

Master some massage therapy. Many experts believe the part of your body that controls hiccups is in the upper part of your spinal column, in the back of your neck. Several of these remedies apply pressure to nerve centers that may be connected to this control site.

- pull gently on your tongue

- massage your earlobes

- with a spoon, lift the uvula (the small tissue hanging down at the back of your throat)

- pinch your upper lip, just below your right nostril

- apply gentle pressure to your closed eyelids

Stimulate your throat. The nerves at the back of your throat can trigger the muscle spasm that's causing your hiccups. By distracting those nerves with something else, you might be able to stop those annoying hiccups.

- sip ice water
- gargle
- swallow some sugar
- bite on a lemon
- drink from the far side of a glass of water

Check your breathing. The idea is to interrupt the hiccup cycle by stopping the flow of oxygen for a short time.

- draw your knees to your chest and wrap your arms around them and squeeze
- hold your breath
- sneeze
- cough
- breathe into a paper bag

High blood pressure

Drop your blood pressure like a rock

How hard does your heart work? For many people, the answer is "too hard," and they don't even know it.

High blood pressure, also called hypertension, sneaks up on you – no symptoms, no signs, no warnings. When you have high blood pressure, your heart is working too hard to pump blood through your arteries.

This silent killer, if left untreated, can lead to heart disease, kidney disease, and stroke. If you don't get your blood pressure checked regularly, you might never know it's too high until it's too late.

Here's how to tell if you're at risk. Blood pressure readings have two numbers. The top number, called systolic blood pressure, measures the force of your blood against your artery walls as your heart beats. The bottom number, called diastolic blood pressure, measures the force between beats.

Recently, the U.S. government changed its definition of high blood pressure. Now, a blood pressure reading of 120/80 or lower is considered normal. Blood pressure from 120/80 to 140/90 is called prehypertension and should be watched or treated. Anything over 140/90 is high blood pressure.

As you get older, your risk of developing high blood pressure skyrockets. Half of all people over age 60 have high blood pressure. If you're black, you might be at even greater risk. Some risk factors, such as age and race, can't be controlled. But you can lose weight and watch what you eat – critical ways to manage this dangerous condition. Add the following items to your diet and give your hardworking heart a rest.

Minerals. Like the Three Musketeers, this trio of minerals – potassium, calcium, and magnesium – join forces to duel with high blood pressure.

- Potassium. This vital mineral leads the charge against high blood pressure. It neutralizes sodium, often the enemy when it comes to controlling your blood pressure, by flushing it out in your urine. Potassium also relaxes your blood vessels, which improves blood flow. Eat more peas, beans, apricots, peaches, bananas, prunes, oranges, spinach, stewed tomatoes, sweet potatoes, avocados, and figs if you want more potassium in your diet.

- Magnesium. This mineral also helps lower blood pressure by relaxing your blood vessels. And it balances the amount of sodium and potassium in your blood cells – less sodium, more potassium. Magnesium-rich foods include whole wheat breads and cereals, broccoli, chard, spinach, okra, oysters, scallops, sea bass, mackerel, beans, nuts, and seeds.

- Calcium. People who get very little calcium in their diet often have high blood pressure. Like potassium, calcium works by helping your body get rid of sodium through your urine. Cheese, milk, yogurt, broccoli, spinach, turnip greens, mackerel, perch, and salmon are good sources of calcium.

Omega-3 fatty acids. Watch out for saturated fats, but remember, some unsaturated fats are good for you. Omega-3 fatty acids, the polyunsaturated type found in fish, can offer help for your high blood pressure.

Most people eat much more omega-6, a polyunsaturated fat found in vegetable oils, than omega-3. Your body converts omega-6 into a substance that constricts your arteries. That makes your heart work harder to pump blood throughout your body, which increases your blood pressure.

Several studies show that eating fish or taking fish oil supplements lowers blood pressure. That's because your body converts omega-3 into a gentler substance that doesn't tighten your arteries as much.

Switching from omega-6 to omega-3 can be an easy way to lower your blood pressure.

You get omega-3 mainly from fatty fish, such as salmon, mackerel, and tuna. Other foods with omega-3 include flaxseed, canola oil, walnuts, wheat germ, and some green leafy vegetables, like collard and turnip greens.

Monounsaturated fat. Further evidence that not all fats are bad comes from olive oil. This staple of the Mediterranean diet contains mostly monounsaturated fat. In a recent study comparing diets rich in olive oil and sunflower oil, a polyunsaturated fat, the olive oil diet drastically lowered blood pressure while the sunflower oil diet only lowered it slightly. The olive oil diet made such a difference that many people on the diet cut in half the amount of blood pressure medication they were taking, under the guidance of their doctors.

Fiber. You already know you should eat fiber-rich foods for protection against heart disease, stroke, and cancer. Well, here's one more reason. A four-year follow-up study found that women who ate more than 25 grams of fiber a day were about 25 percent less likely to develop high blood pressure as women who ate less than 10 grams of fiber every day.

Fruits, vegetables, and whole-grain breads and cereals are good sources of fiber. For example, one potato with skin has 5 grams of fiber, an orange has 3 grams, and a cup of raisin bran has 8 grams. Fiber works best over the long term. Don't get discouraged if your blood pressure doesn't drop right away.

Garlic. This fragrant herb does more than add flavor to meals. It also lowers cholesterol and protects your arteries from clogging. That way, your blood can zip through with less "oomph" from your heart. Some studies show garlic lowers your systolic blood pressure by nearly 7 percent and your diastolic blood pressure by almost 8 percent. Try garlic's cousin, the onion, as another tasty cooking alternatives to salt.

Celery to the rescue

If you went to an Asian herbalist asking for advice about high blood pressure, chances are he'd tell you to take four stalks of celery daily and call him in a week.

Experts say the crunchy vegetable contains a chemical that can lower levels of stress hormones in your blood. This allows blood vessels to expand, giving your blood more room and reducing pressure. Munch on this tasty veggie every day and watch your blood pressure go down.

DASH high blood pressure in 2 weeks

Be careful what you put on your plate. Your eating habits can contribute to the development of high blood pressure. Luckily, researchers have found an eating plan that can reduce high blood pressure in as little as two weeks.

A scientific study called "DASH" (Dietary Approaches to Stop Hypertension) found that high blood pressure was reduced when people ate less saturated fat, total fat, and cholesterol and more fruits, vegetables, and low-fat dairy foods.

The researchers compared three eating plans:

- A typical American diet

- A diet similar to the first but with more fruits and vegetables

- The DASH diet – low in saturated fat, total fat, and cholesterol and rich in fruits, vegetables, and low-fat dairy foods

People on the DASH diet reduced their systolic blood pressure an average of six points and their diastolic blood pressure an average of three points.

In the people who had high blood pressure, systolic dropped by 11 points and diastolic dropped by six points. This reduction occurred within just two weeks of starting the diet. The really good news is that the DASH diet isn't hard to follow.

The National Heart, Lung, and Blood Institute offers these tips for beginning the DASH plan.

- Change gradually. If you now eat one or two vegetables a day, add a serving at lunch and another at dinner.

- If you don't eat fruit now or have only juice at breakfast, add a serving to your meals or have it as a snack.

- Use half the butter, margarine, or salad dressing you do now.

- Try low-fat or fat-free condiments, such as mayonnaise and salad dressings.

- Gradually increase dairy products to three servings every day. For example, drink milk with lunch or dinner instead of soda or sugar-sweetened tea. Choose low-fat (1 percent) or fat-free (skim) dairy products to reduce your total fat intake.

- Limit meat, poultry, and fish to two 3-ounce servings a day or less. A 3-ounce serving is about the size of a deck of cards.

- If you now eat large portions of meat, cut back gradually by a half or a third at each meal. Treat meat as one part of the whole meal, instead of the focus.

- Include two or more vegetarian meals each week.

- Increase servings of vegetables, rice, pasta, and dry beans in your meals.

- Try casseroles, pasta, and stir-fry dishes with less meat and more vegetables, grains, and dry beans.

■ Use fruits or low-fat foods as desserts and snacks. Buy fruits canned in their own juice. Fresh fruits require little or no preparation. Dried fruits are easy to carry with you.

■ Try these snack ideas – unsalted pretzels or nuts mixed with raisins, graham crackers, low-fat and fat-free yogurt and frozen yogurt, plain popcorn with no salt or butter added, and raw vegetables, like celery and carrots.

Because the DASH diet has more daily servings of fruits, vegetables, and grains than most people are used to, the increase in fiber could cause bloating and diarrhea.

To avoid this discomfort, increase your servings of fruits, vegetables, and grains gradually. Although you may see results in just two weeks, the DASH diet is really an eating plan for life. You must change your eating habits permanently if you want to maintain lower blood pressure.

For more information, visit the National Heart, Lung, and Blood Institute's Web site <www.nhlbi.nih.gov> or write to them at: NHLBI Health Information Center, P.O. Box 30105, Bethesda, MD 20824-0105.

'C' how orange juice can help

Lower your blood pressure naturally and put the spring back in your arteries – with orange juice.

In a recent study, people with high blood pressure who took a 500-milligram (mg) supplement of vitamin C each day for a month reduced their blood pressure by almost 10 percent. People in the study who took a placebo also reduced their blood pressure, but only by about 3 percent.

Another study found that after people took vitamin C, their arteries became significantly less stiff, and their platelets were less sticky, reducing the risk of blood clots. The people taking a placebo experienced no change.

Vitamin C is a potent antioxidant, and researchers believe it protects your body's supply of nitric oxide, which helps blood vessels relax.

While more research is needed to confirm these findings, most people would benefit by eating foods rich in vitamin C. Along with orange juice, citrus fruits, strawberries, sweet red peppers, and green peppers are excellent sources.

Toss your blood pressure pills for good

Blood pressure drugs have undoubtedly prevented many deaths from heart disease and stroke in the last 30 years. According to a recent study, however, some people could do just as well without the drugs – if they're willing to make a few lifestyle changes. Doctors sometimes prescribe medication to people with mild high blood pressure simply because they know most people won't follow their diet and exercise advice.

If you only take one drug to treat mild high blood pressure, you may be able to stop buying those expensive little pills. Instead, you'll have to make lifestyle changes, such as maintaining an ideal body weight and following a low-salt, low-alcohol diet. Of course, you should never stop taking any prescription drug without your doctor's approval. But if you would like to try lowering your blood pressure naturally, talk with him about these drug-free methods. Then, with his approval, try them.

Discover the Mediterranean way. Eat less fat, the experts say. But you can have your fat – within reason – and lower your blood pressure, too, if you eat like they do in Greece and southern Italy. A recent study found that people who replaced some of the saturated fat, like cream, butter, and cheese, in their diets with extra-virgin olive oil lowered their blood pressure significantly. Some were able to cut down on their blood pressure medicine or stop taking it altogether.

According to the American Institute of Cancer Research, olive oil is only one part of healthy eating in that part of the world. People in the Mediterranean eat a huge variety of plants, so much so that the people of Crete were once called "mangifolia," which means "leaf-eaters." They also eat very little red meat or packaged foods, plenty of fish and vegetables, and drink a little red wine.

Because variety is an important part of their diet, they eat small portions of many foods every day. The abundance of plant foods contributes lots of natural fiber, which has been linked to successful weight loss and good health. Who said a heart-healthy diet has to be boring?

Eat less, move more. Eating right is only half the battle when it comes to lowering blood pressure. Exercise provides the other half. A recent study found that a diet and exercise program not only lowered blood pressure, but also helped maintain that lower reading during times of mental stress.

Losing as little as 3 percent of your body weight can help lower your blood pressure. If you weigh 200 pounds, you could have lower blood pressure after losing only six pounds. But why stop there? Keep going until you reach your ideal weight.

Once your doctor clears you for exercise, get started right away. Try brisk walking if you haven't exercised in a while. As you tone up and slim down, you can ask your doctor about swimming, bicycling, and other forms of exercise.

Give up salt. While scientists disagree on whether a low-salt diet can lower blood pressure for everyone, you're probably getting a lot more of this mineral than you need. Try skimping on the salt for a while. If it turns out you're salt sensitive, your blood pressure should go down.

Shake off bad habits. If you're worried about developing high blood pressure, you can make some lifestyle changes to decrease your risk. Don't smoke, and if you drink, limit your alcohol. That means no more than two drinks a day for a man, and one drink a day for a woman.

If you can manage to control your blood pressure without drugs, you'll save money and avoid unwanted side effects. Nevertheless, if you need to take medicine, don't hesitate. High blood pressure can have deadly results, and new research shows it even affects your thinking skills.

A sharp mind depends on a steady supply of oxygen-rich blood. Untreated high blood pressure can damage the inside of your arteries, hindering blood flow. To increase your powers of memory and concentration, work with your doctor to keep your blood pressure under control.

Beware of the 'grapefruit effect'

If you're taking medicine for your high blood pressure, be careful what you wash it down with. Grapefruit juice in the morning may be nutritious and delicious, but it could cause your blood pressure medication to build up to toxic levels in your body. The "grapefruit effect" on drugs was discovered accidentally by researchers several years ago when they gave volunteers grapefruit juice to hide the taste of a drug. They found out that when the medicine was taken with grapefruit juice, it multiplied the amount of the medication in the blood.

Later studies found that grapefruit contains a substance that blocks the effects of an enzyme, which helps break down certain types of drugs in your body. Instead of being metabolized, the drugs continue to circulate in your body and can accumulate to dangerous levels.

Although the grapefruit effect could help make some drugs more effective, consider the American Heart Association's recommendation – don't drink grapefruit juice at the same time as taking calcium channel blockers.

Other drugs that may be affected by grapefruit juice include some types of sleeping pills, antihistamines, and cyclosporine. To be sure, ask your doctor or pharmacist if grapefruit juice will affect your medication.

High cholesterol

4 unbeatable ways to lower your cholesterol

You think you're as healthy as a horse – until the doctor's office calls with the results of your physical, and you find out your cholesterol is pushing 300. A high cholesterol level is a warning that your heart is headed for trouble, but you can do something about it.

Snack to your heart's content. Don't be afraid to snack several times a day on low-fat foods, such as yogurt, fruit, vegetables, bagels, and whole-grain breads and cereals. As a matter of fact, evidence points to lower cholesterol levels in people who eat small meals throughout the day instead of three large meals. Eating often keeps hormones, like insulin, from rising and signaling your body to make cholesterol. Just make sure your total intake of calories doesn't go up when you eat more often.

Eat less saturated fat. You get cholesterol two ways. Your body manufactures most of it in your liver, but you get dietary cholesterol from animal products, such as meat, milk, cheese, butter, and eggs. Plant foods, like fruits, vegetables, grains, and nuts, don't have any cholesterol.

While eating less cholesterol may help, the biggest dietary change you can make is to reduce your intake of saturated fat. Too much saturated fat can raise your cholesterol levels. Animal fats, like butter and lard, and some vegetable fats, like palm oil and coconut oil, are saturated. Substituting a liquid vegetable oil, like canola, when you're cooking is a good way to lower saturated fat in your diet.

Here's a general guideline – the more saturated a fat is, the more solid it is at room temperature. You don't have to cut fat out of your diet altogether. Researchers say moderate decreases in fat intake can substantially lower cholesterol.

Get some exercise. Exercise can help you increase your good HDL cholesterol level and lower your bad LDL cholesterol. It also helps you lose weight and control diabetes and high blood pressure. And when you exercise, you are conditioning your heart along with your other muscles. All that adds up to good news for your heart.

Maintain a healthy weight. If you are overweight, lose weight. Weight loss lowers triglycerides and LDL cholesterol and raises HDL cholesterol. Researchers found that losing weight can increase your HDL cholesterol regardless of how much you exercise. If you exercise and lose weight, you will increase your HDL even more.

How to tame bad cholesterol

Need another reason to keep piling spinach and carrots on your dinner plate? Try lutein, a pigment found in green and yellow vegetables. Studies have already proven this nutrient is important for your eyes. Now research at the University of Southern California in Los Angeles shows it's good for your heart as well.

The study followed 480 middle-age men and women for 18 months. During that time, those who had the most lutein in their bloodstream had almost no increase in the thickness of their carotid (neck) arteries.

This was a good sign that the bad LDL cholesterol had not oxidized inside them and formed the dangerous plaque that can lead to heart attacks. Results of two other parts of the study, one done in the lab with human tissue and the other with mice, supported the findings of the first.

Dr. James Dwyer, who led this research, recommends eating plenty of lutein-rich foods to keep your arteries clear. "A diet rich in vegetables, including the dark green leafy variety," he says, "will provide sufficient lutein to achieve the levels of persons in our study."

Dwyer recommends at least one serving a day of foods like spinach, kale, collard greens, turnip greens, romaine lettuce, broccoli, zucchini squash, corn, brussels sprouts, and peas.

But he suggests you bypass the lutein supplements. The benefits of nutrients found in supplements, he points out, aren't always the same as those you get in foods and can even be risky.

"For example," he says, "vegetables rich in beta carotene are probably protective against some cancers, but beta carotene supplements are toxic and increase the risk of lung cancer." Since the risks of lutein supplements haven't been determined yet, he suggests you stick to the vegetables.

Some doctors may advise those with kidney problems to avoid large quantities of leafy dark greens, Dwyer notes. But he doesn't think the research supports the fear these vegetables might increase kidney stones.

Lutein is just one way to protect your heart. Here are some additional nutrients that will help keep your cholesterol in check and aid in your fight against a number of other diseases as well.

Fiber. When it comes to lowering cholesterol and protecting your heart, saturated fat is the enemy and fiber is a hero. Fiber slashes LDL cholesterol while leaving the good HDL cholesterol alone. One six-year study involving more than 40,000 men found that, for every additional 10 grams of cereal fiber the men ate, their risk of heart disease decreased by an astounding 29 percent.

High-fiber foods are also more filling, which can help you lose weight and lower your risk of heart disease even more. To get lots of fiber, eat whole grains and fresh fruits and vegetables.

Magnesium. According to experts, most people get less than half the magnesium they need daily, and the consequences can be dangerous. Studies have linked magnesium deficiency to increased cancer risk, especially esophageal cancer. Adding this mineral to your diet could lower your cholesterol by as much as 33 percent. One study found that giving magnesium to people immediately after a severe heart attack cut their death rate in half during the critical four weeks following the attacks, when compared to heart attack victims who didn't get magnesium.

The recommended dietary allowance (RDA) for magnesium is 420 milligrams (mg) for men over 30 and 320 mg for women over 30. To reach this level, eat at least five servings of fresh or minimally processed fruits and vegetables daily. Avocados, sunflower seeds, pinto beans, spinach, oysters, and broccoli are especially good sources of this mineral.

Vitamin E. This fat-soluble vitamin may not lower cholesterol levels, but, like lutein, it can prevent LDL cholesterol from becoming oxidized and sticking to your artery walls.

In one study, men who took at least 100 international units (IU) of vitamin E daily for at least two years had 37 percent fewer heart attacks than men who didn't take supplements. And a separate study found that women who took vitamin E supplements had 41 percent fewer heart attacks.

The RDA for vitamin E is 22 IU or 15 mg. However, most studies that show a benefit to taking supplements used doses between 100 and 400 IU daily. Be sure to check with your doctor before taking more than the RDA of vitamin E, especially if you're taking blood-thinning medication. Good food sources of vitamin E include wheat germ oil, sunflower seeds, peanuts, mangoes, sweet potatoes, and olive oil.

Vitamin C. This is another antioxidant vitamin that helps prevent LDL cholesterol from becoming oxidized, and studies show it also helps raise HDL cholesterol levels.

Unlike vitamin E, however, vitamin C is a water-soluble vitamin, which means it isn't stored by your body. That makes it even more important to get as much of it as you need every day. Fortunately, that isn't difficult. Just one cup of orange juice gives you more than the RDA. Other good sources include sweet red peppers, green peppers, cantaloupe, brussels sprouts, grapefruit, and tomato juice.

Niacin. This B vitamin works so well to lower cholesterol, doctors prescribe it as a treatment. However, high doses can cause itching, flushing, rash, and stomach pain as well as more serious side effects such as ulcers, liver damage, and symptoms of diabetes. To get your niacin naturally, eat tuna, chicken, liver, salmon, potatoes, and beans.

Spread the good news about fake fats

You may love buttered toast for breakfast, but you know it's not exactly a heart-healthy way to start your day. Of course, choosing whole-grain bread will give you a good dose of cholesterol-lowering fiber, but butter is high in saturated fat, and a pat of trans-fatty margarine could be even worse.

Fortunately, your supermarket dairy case holds several healthy alternatives, according to the National Institutes of Health (NIH). Instead of butter or margarine, choose Benecol Spread, a fat substitute endorsed by the Food and Drug Administration (FDA) for its cholesterol-lowering ability. Or try Take Control, another spread that gives you the same heart-healthy benefits.

New NIH guidelines for lowering cholesterol recommend 2 grams of plant stanols, found in Benecol, or sterols, found in Take Control, every day. Both substances work by blocking your body's absorption of cholesterol. As a bonus, they also help prevent certain cancers, including colon, breast, ovarian, and prostate cancers. Read the label to see how much of the spread you'll need to get the suggested amount.

Other fat substitutes allow you to enjoy an occasional high-fat snack without worrying that your cholesterol level will skyrocket. Olestra, for example, takes potato chips off the high-danger list. It can't increase your cholesterol because your body won't digest it, but it may cause some unpleasant side effects in your intestinal tract. And chips, no matter what they're made of, aren't particularly healthy, so think twice before using them to replace nutritious snacks like fruit.

Hydrogenated oils, used by the ton in fast-food restaurants, are guaranteed to harden your arteries. Once again, a product has come to the rescue that makes fried foods a little safer to eat. Appetize is a blend of corn oil and beef tallow with the natural cholesterol removed. Some research suggests it also might help lower blood cholesterol.

Unfortunately, fast-food restaurants aren't rushing to replace their artery-clogging fats with this substitute. Until they do, go easy on the burgers and fries, and try to eat more meals at home where you can take advantage of healthy fat substitutes.

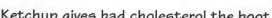

Ketchup gives bad cholesterol the boot

A hot dog might not do your heart any favors, but what you put on top just might. Some studies have shown that lycopene, which is found naturally in tomatoes, can lower your risk of heart disease and certain types of cancer. But according to a recent study, the best source of lycopene is not tomatoes, it's ketchup.

Research funded by the H.J. Heinz food company and endorsed by the Cancer Research Foundation of America reveals that cooked tomatoes, like those used to make ketchup, provide as much as five times more lycopene than fresh tomatoes.

This natural antioxidant protects your heart by preventing the oxidation of bad LDL cholesterol in your arteries. Lycopene doesn't lessen the amount of cholesterol in your blood. It just keeps the cholesterol from doing any damage.

In a Canadian study at the University of Toronto, people were given one-to-two servings a day of tomato-based products, such as tomato juice, spaghetti sauce, and concentrated lycopene.

After just one week, lycopene levels were doubled in the study participants and their levels of oxidized LDL cholesterol went down significantly.

So how much ketchup do you need to reap these great benefits? Getting about 40 milligrams (mg) of lycopene a day is enough to give you a leg up in the fight against heart disease. Unfortunately, you'd have to drown your hot dog in about a cup of ketchup to get this much.

But there are other ways to get lycopene. Almost anything tomato-based is a rich source. Just two cups of tomato juice or 3/4 cup of spaghetti sauce will do the trick. You can also get lycopene from guava, watermelon, and pink grapefruit.

Develop an appreciation for artichokes

Don't let this prickly, unusual-looking vegetable intimidate you. If you've never cooked or eaten an artichoke, now is the time to try this vitamin-packed, heart-healthy treat.

You can buy whole, fresh artichokes or hearts and crowns that are canned or frozen. The whole artichoke is fun and easy to eat. What you buy in the store is actually the flower bud of the artichoke plant, which has been harvested by hand. When you get your artichoke home, simply wash it, cut off the stem, and pull off the bottom, outer layer of petals.

Usually, whole artichokes are either steamed or boiled, but don't forget your microwave. If you cook it in a little bit of water, lemon juice, and olive oil, you may find the flavor so good you don't need a sauce.

After cooking, simply pull the petals off, one by one, and eat the soft lining. Eventually, you'll get to the heart, which is entirely edible and has a great nutty flavor. Because of their flavor and nutrients, artichoke hearts are becoming increasingly popular in stir-fries, pasta dishes, and casseroles.

One medium-size artichoke gives you a quarter of your daily fiber needs. In addition, it is extremely high in vitamin C, potassium, folic acid, magnesium, and other important minerals. And unless you dip it in butter, the artichoke is fat-free and low in calories.

There's another good reason to become an artichoke lover – to lower your cholesterol. In one study, people with high cholesterol received artichoke juice instead of cholesterol-lowering drugs. Their bad LDL cholesterol, total cholesterol, and triglyceride levels fell an average of 8 percent, while their good HDL cholesterol levels increased. The people taking traditional medicines lowered their cholesterol levels only a few percentage points more.

Other researchers have noticed that artichokes improve blood fat levels overall. It seems that something in the artichoke stimulates the liver into producing more bile. The bile grabs fat molecules, allowing the enzymes in the intestines to digest them. More bile means less fat in your bloodstream.

The next time you're at the grocery store toss an artichoke in your cart and make your heart happy.

Impotence

Take impotence to heart

They say the way to a man's heart is through his stomach – but women have always suspected it lies a little bit lower. Turns out both areas have important links to the heart as well as to each other. Read on to discover the relationship between love handles, impotence, and atherosclerosis – and how to firm up your defense against this potentially deadly condition.

Be alert to the heart disease link. Viagra has given many men a second lease on life. Besides its obvious benefit, the impotence drug has an added bonus of helping doctors discover heart disease in its early stages. Because of Viagra's possible harmful effects on the heart, men often visit a cardiologist to make sure they can safely take the drug.

Dr. Marc R. Pritzker of the Minneapolis Heart Institute Foundation recently tested 50 men between the ages of 40 and 65 who had trouble getting or maintaining an erection. A whopping 80 percent of them had more than one risk factor for heart disease, including high blood pressure, high cholesterol, smoking, and a sedentary lifestyle. And 40 percent had serious blockages of their heart arteries.

"We now understand that atherosclerosis detected in one set of blood vessels markedly increases the chances of having this form of blood vessel disease in other areas of the body, including the heart, brain, legs and kidneys," Pritzker explains.

"Because the blood vessels that supply the penis are narrower than arteries in other areas of the body, atherosclerosis – the disease process that leads to heart attacks and strokes – may manifest itself as erectile dysfunction before the disease becomes apparent in other arteries."

Other studies have reached similar conclusions. A trial by Dr. Kevin Billups of St. Paul, Minn., found that 60 percent of the 57 impotent men studied had high cholesterol. Of that group, 91 percent also showed signs of arterial disease after experiencing impotence problems.

Of course, just because you have impotence doesn't mean you have atherosclerosis. It could be a side effect of medication, depression, stress, or fatigue, or even a psychological problem. But Pritzker estimates atherosclerosis is to blame in up to 50 percent of all impotence cases.

"A man having regular sexual activity who experiences a consistent change in erectile function may be demonstrating signs of atherosclerosis where arteries become clogged and the heart muscle does not receive enough blood," he says.

"As we become more thorough in our questioning of patients, it is not uncommon to hear that erectile dysfunction preceded the onset of heart disease by a year or more. Thus erectile dysfunction may be an early warning sign of the potential for heart problems."

If you're experiencing trouble with erections, you may want to schedule an appointment with a cardiologist and have him screen you for coronary artery disease.

Trim your belly to trim your risk. Before you buy a bigger pair of pants, remember your risk of impotence expands along with your waistline.

Harvard professor Eric B. Rimm recently led a study that determined waist size had a big impact on erectile dysfunction. For example, a man with a 42-inch waist was nearly twice as likely to experience impotence as a man with a 32-inch waist.

Rimm and colleagues also found men who exercised 30 minutes a day were 41 percent less likely to be impotent than those who engaged in the least amount of exercise.

These results make sense, considering obesity and a sedentary life-style are also risk factors for atherosclerosis.

You should begin to see a definite link – a big belly is a risk factor for impotence, which might be a sign of atherosclerosis, which might be caused by a big belly.

If that sounds too confusing, just remember that the risk factors for impotence and atherosclerosis are the same.

Prevent two problems at once. Because of the close relationship between impotence and atherosclerosis, the steps you take to prevent one also help you guard against the other.

Here are a few simple, healthy lifestyle changes you can make to combat both impotence and atherosclerosis.

- Exercise. Even if you start late in life, exercise is the most effective way to lower your risk for impotence. So get moving and exercise every day.

- Eat a healthy diet. Cut down on salt and saturated fat, found mainly in meat, eggs, dairy products, and hydrogenated vegetable oils, and eat more fruits, vegetables, and whole grains. That way, you'll help keep your weight, blood pressure, and cholesterol under control.

- Drink moderately. Rimm's study found that men who had one or two drinks a day cut their risk for impotence by one-third compared to men who drank alcohol more often or not at all.

- Stop smoking. You'll do wonders for your arteries – and your overall health.

Sometimes, a few changes are all it takes to save your heart and your sex life. According to Pritzker, "The heart disease found in the study participants was treatable, and in many cases, the men's erectile dysfunction went away when they quit smoking or got their cholesterol levels under control."

Cure impotence with pelvic exercises

Just as you have muscles that allow you to walk, talk, and breathe, you have muscles that affect your ability to achieve and maintain an erection. In many cases, getting these muscles back into shape can eliminate impotence once and for all.

Pelvic muscle exercises, called Kegels, are designed to help you do just that. Women have been practicing them for years to help firm vaginal muscles, particularly after childbirth.

Now researchers have found that these exercises help men as well. This routine developed by therapists at Boston's Beth Israel Hospital can help you regain control of your sex life.

■ Squeeze your pelvic muscles as if you're trying to stop a flow of urine. You should feel your anal pelvic muscles contract also. Hold for 10 seconds, then relax for 10 seconds.

■ Repeat this cycle up to 15 times, or until you can no longer hold the flex for a full 10 seconds.

■ Take a few minutes to relax.

■ Now do a fast set. Squeeze for a second and relax for a second, 10 times in a row.

■ Do 10 sets of these, resting between sets.

You can perform these exercises as often as you like or as often as your doctor says you can. Be patient and stick with the program, and you should begin to see benefits before long.

Kegels can also be used to combat another frustrating problem, urinary incontinence. Follow the same steps listed above, but add this extra technique.

■ When urinating, use your pelvic muscles to stop the flow of urine in mid-stream. Repeat this exercise several times until your bladder is empty.

If you do this every time you urinate, the extra practice will help strengthen your muscles. During situations that cause leakage, constrict your pelvic muscles just as you do when practicing Kegels. Pretty soon, you'll be able to prevent most accidents just by squeezing your new, stronger muscles.

Latest way to sidestep bicycle-seat injuries

Bicycling is a great aerobic exercise, but you may be sitting on a hidden danger. Several studies show that bicycle seats can cause impotence; perineal (area between the anus and scrotum) numbness; and injuries to blood vessels, nerves, and other delicate tissue.

In a European study of long-distance male cyclists, 22 percent of the riders reported penile numbness and 13 percent reported impotence. In another study, 41 percent of weekend bike riders reported impotence. Surprisingly, 20 percent of riders of stationary exercise bikes suffered impotence, too.

Damage can occur when a narrow bike seat focuses your body's weight on the arteries and nerves that supply the pubic region. And for long-distance cyclists, that pressure may be exerted for long periods of time, increasing the risk of damage.

Problems with bikes aren't limited to men. At the American Urological Association in May 1999, several studies were presented that suggested possible perineal injury from bicycling in both men and women.

Researchers at Boston University studied 282 female bikers ages 18 to 76. Of these women, 32 percent reported injuries from bicycle top tubes (the horizontal bar just below the seat) and 34 percent reported perineal numbness.

Biking injuries can also cause urinary tract problems. But don't put your bicycle up for sale just yet. Bicycling is a healthy and enjoyable activity.

Here are some simple steps you can take to lessen your risk of common bicycle-seat injuries.

■ Switch to a recumbent bike. You're seated lower on these bikes, and you lean back, with your back against a support. This means your weight is more evenly distributed.

■ Get a new, ergonomic bike seat with a cut out area that completely takes the pressure off delicate nerves and arteries. These are available for about $50 in styles for men and women. Just visit your local bicycle shop.

■ Get a wider bicycle seat, allowing your weight to be distributed more evenly.

■ Rise out of your seat every 10 minutes and pedal for several minutes in a standing position.

■ Change position frequently while riding.

■ Adjust the handlebars and the height of your seat, making it horizontal or even pointing downward to take the pressure off. A knowledgeable employee in a bike shop can do this for you.

Insomnia

Natural solutions for sleepless nights

If you've been tossing and turning more than you've been snoozing lately, you may be tempted to reach for some over-the-counter sleeping pills. Before you do, give these natural solutions a try.

Stick to a schedule. Have a regular time to settle down for the night to establish a rhythm to help trigger sleep. And get up at the same time every morning, even on weekends.

Take time to relax before bed. Take about 30 minutes before bedtime to relax and wind down. Read a good book, take a warm bath, or work on a hobby. Low lights and soft music can help get you in the mood for sleep. Avoid watching intense television shows or dealing with unpleasant tasks during your wind-down time. That way you'll be calm, cool, and collected when you get into bed.

Get cozy. It's much easier to fall asleep if you're comfortable. Start with a good mattress and pillow and wear comfortable clothes to bed. Make sure your room is quiet and dark and keep the temperature at whatever is most comfortable for you.

Don't push it. You can't force yourself to sleep. If you've been lying in bed staring at the ceiling for more than a half hour, get up. Try to do some quiet activities, and then go back to bed.

Use your bed for sleep only. Going to bed should signal your body that it's time to sleep. If you watch television, work, or eat in bed, your body may get confused and won't automatically relax for sleep like it should.

Warm your toes. If you have cold hands and feet, you might benefit from using a hot water bottle or wearing socks when you first go to bed. Warming your hands and feet and then removing the socks or hot water bottle helps your blood vessels dilate. Research indicates that blood vessel dilation in your feet and hands is an important step in falling asleep.

Exercise. About 20 to 30 minutes of exercise three or four days a week could improve your sleep – but timing is important. Exercise too close to bedtime can be stimulating rather than relaxing.

Drink warm milk. Warm milk has been a home remedy for insomnia for years. Milk contains tryptophan, an amino acid that researchers say can help you sleep. It's also high in calcium and magnesium, two minerals that are important in producing melatonin, which controls your sleep cycle.

Give up caffeine and nicotine. If you depend on coffee to wake you up in the morning, remember it can also keep you up at night. Limit your intake of coffee, tea, colas, and other drinks containing caffeine, especially in the evening. Caffeine is a stimulant, but you may not realize that nicotine in cigarettes is a stimulant, too.

Ditch the alcohol. You may think that a beer or a glass of wine before bed will relax you and help you fall asleep. It may – but it usually results in wakefulness later on in the night. If you really want to sleep tight, don't drink alcohol in the evening.

Get some morning sun. You'll sleep better at night if you soak up some bright light early in the day. Morning sunshine increases the level of melatonin in your body. This hormone helps regulate your sleep cycle naturally.

Keep your tummy content. Going to bed hungry can keep you awake, but eating a heavy meal before bedtime isn't a good idea either. A busy digestive system can interfere with sleep.

Try valerian. This herb has been used for over 1,000 years as a mild sedative and sleep aid. It is particularly popular in Europe, and the German Commission E has approved it as a calmative and sleep-promoting product. Valerian does not interact with alcohol, and it's remarkably free of side effects. For a relaxing cup of valerian tea, add two teaspoons of dried root to a cup of hot water.

Practice gradual relaxation. If you are too tense to sleep, try relaxing your muscles, one group at a time. Beginning with your toes, work your way up – feet, calves, thighs, abdomen, hips, and so forth – until you reach your scalp. By that point, you should be relaxed and ready for sleep.

Eat some cherries. Have trouble sleeping? Cherries might be your key to dreamland. Dr. Russel Reiter of the University of Texas Health Science Center recently discovered that cherries contain large amounts of melatonin, a hormone that helps you sleep. "Certainly, cherries to this point have the highest concentration of melatonin we've measured in any fruit," Reiter says. Melatonin works either as a direct sleep-inducing substance or by opening what Reiter calls "the sleep gate," which puts you in the right frame of mind to sleep. Eating cherries just before bedtime would give you the most benefit.

Because it's an antioxidant, melatonin can also neutralize free radicals that contribute to cancer, Alzheimer's disease, and signs of aging, like crow's feet around your eyes. Although research is still in the early stages, scientists think you may get all the melatonin you need by eating just a handful of cherries a day. Eating cherries might be especially important if you're older because as you age, your body doesn't produce as much melatonin on its own.

Better sleep = better waistline

Don't have the energy to do endless sit-ups and crunches to flatten your jelly belly? Maybe what you really need is a good night's sleep. According to a recent study, people treated for sleep apnea (a disorder in which you stop breathing for brief periods during sleep) lost abdominal fat, although they didn't necessarily lose weight. Volunteers not treated for their apnea had no change in fat distribution.

The researchers think it's possible the people lost fat because more sleep altered their metabolism favorably. Or it could be they simply had more energy to burn fat during the day after a good night's sleep.

Either way, if you suffer from sleep apnea, or anything that could be interfering with your sleep, get it treated. You'll gain a good night's sleep and perhaps lose some inches around your middle.

Put these tricks to the test

If you're desperate for a peaceful snooze and haven't found anything that helps, you might try a few of these unusual ideas. They may seem weird, but at least one person swears by each of them.

■ Sleep with a pillow over your head but not over your face.

■ Wear a hat to bed. (This person may have gotten the idea from the children's book, *Miss Twiggley's Tree*. Funny Miss Twiggley lived in a tree and slept in her hat.)

■ Read something really boring like a psychological, or other technical, journal article.

■ Imagine you are a cat and stretch like one. Extend your legs and arms as far as possible for about 15 minutes. Purr if the mood strikes you.

■ Sleep in a cold room. In summer, turn the air down to about 60 degrees. If you let the cold air hit your feet, you may cool down faster. In the winter, leave your bedroom windows open about 1 to 2 inches to let the cold air in.

- Imagine driving down a highway. Pretend you see a billboard ahead with the word "SLEEP" on it.

- Sniff some chopped onion. Keep it in a jar beside your bed. Open it and smell it at bedtime. You should be asleep in about 15 minutes.

- Give yourself a stomach massage. Start at your navel and make gentle circles with your hand in a clockwise direction. Make your circles bigger and bigger until you reach the outside of your stomach. Then make gradually smaller circles going back to the navel. Do it again in a counter-clockwise direction. Repeat the whole process with the other hand.

- Try gently rocking your body like you would rock a baby while sitting in a straight chair, not a rocking chair. The motion is from side to side, rather than back and forth. You may find this motion very relaxing.

- Get someone to pay you to sleep. In a study at a sleep center in England, people who were paid actually fell asleep faster.

- Visualize the details of a peaceful, calming scene. When you've really got it clear in your mind, imagine a comfortable spot to lie down. Curl up and go to sleep.

- If all else fails, go back to the old stand-by – counting sheep, old sweethearts, the number of cars you hear passing, your breaths, anything that will bore you into sleep.

Spring forward safely

With springtime comes daylight savings time and an extra hour you can spend outside at the end of the day. You may enjoy planting flowers, tossing a frisbee, or just catching up on neighborhood news.

Unfortunately, this bright picture has a dark side. During the first few days of daylight savings time, you are more likely to have a traffic accident.

A Canadian study reported in *The New England Journal of Medicine* found about 8 percent more traffic accidents on the first Monday after the spring time change. Drivers were less alert because they lost one hour of sleep.

Avoiding this problem seems simple enough. On the night when daylight savings time goes into effect, just go to bed an hour earlier and wake up an hour earlier. It's the same amount of sleep, right?

Sadly, it just doesn't work that smoothly. Researchers say it takes about five days for your body clock to fully adjust to the time change.

The best way to prepare for a safe "spring forward" is to ease forward. Start adjusting your sleep time a week before the start of daylight savings time.

Set your alarm clock for 10 minutes earlier each morning and go to bed 10 minutes earlier each night. Your body clock should accept this gradual adjustment more readily.

Fortunately, when fall comes, researchers find a drop in accidents equal to the increase in spring.

Irritable bowel syndrome

8 ways to soothe a 'cranky' bowel

It's one of the leading causes of employee absenteeism in the United States, and yet many people don't even know what it is, partly because most people are too embarrassed to discuss it.

Irritable bowel syndrome (IBS) is also known as "spastic colon" or "irritable colon," and is actually a set of chronic digestive symptoms. IBS symptoms include abdominal pain, frequent constipation and/or diarrhea, cramping, gas, and sometimes bloating, nausea, headache, and fatigue.

IBS affects more women than men, and symptoms usually begin in your 20s or 30s. It seldom begins after age 55. IBS isn't life-threatening, but it can make your life more difficult. Luckily, it can be controlled with a few diet and lifestyle changes.

Slow down. Everyone seems to be in a hurry these days, so mealtime may be a short affair. Unfortunately, gulping down your food increases the chances you'll gulp air, too. That's a good reason to slow down and enjoy your food.

Steer clear of gas producers. Certain foods are more likely to cause you to have gas, which can aggravate your IBS. Limit your intake of beans, cabbage, onions, or any other food that has a tendency to make you react this way.

Can the carbonated drinks. Sodas and other carbonated drinks can also increase gas in your intestines, so limit your intake of those, too.

Manage your stress. By reducing the stress in your life, you can give your digestive system a much-needed break. Your system is sensitive to stress, and many experts believe stress and activities that tax your body are particularly harsh on your bowels. Try exercise or meditation to help manage your IBS symptoms.

Dodge the dairy. Although it may not affect you, lactose intolerance bothers about 40 percent of people with IBS. Look for ways to cut down on dairy products. Today, lactose-free products are being developed from such items as soy, rice, and even almonds.

Choose the right fiber. Fiber is essential to staying regular, but research suggests that bran and other grains may actually make IBS worse. Instead, try getting your fiber from gentler sources, such as fruits and cooked vegetables. Researchers have found that these produce better results with far less chance of abdominal pain and bowel disturbance.

Psyllium, the dried seed husks of a certain type of plantain, is another natural way to help regulate yourself. It can be found in such over-the-counter products as Metamucil.

Keep a food diary. People with IBS may be more sensitive to certain foods. A good way to determine what foods cause flare-ups is to keep an IBS journal. When you experience symptoms, record what you have eaten recently, as well as your activities and any stress you may be under. By keeping such a journal, you may see patterns forming and can prevent further outbreaks by avoiding their causes.

Try a little peppermint. For a natural way to relieve your bowel discomfort, try some peppermint oil. It may relax your intestinal muscles and soothe your cramps. If you take it as an enteric-coated capsule, it will dissolve in the intestines rather than the stomach, where it can irritate your stomach lining. Some IBS sufferers find relief by taking one to two 0.2 milliliter (ml) capsules three times a day, between meals.

Kidney stones

Action plan prevents kidney stones

Think of kidney stones as a crime. To solve it, first you round up the usual suspects. These include low fluid intake and a high-oxalate diet. If you don't get enough fluids, your urine becomes more concentrated, leading to crystals. Too many crystals can lead to stone formation.

Foods high in oxalate include beets, rhubarb, strawberries, nuts, chocolate, spinach, and other green leafy vegetables. Other possible suspects include a low-calcium diet, which causes your body to absorb more oxalate, and a diet high in salt. Also take family history into account.

"The best advice is to maintain a high fluid intake, aiming for half water, with a goal of keeping very little color to the urine," says Dr. Richard W. Norman, professor and head of the urology department at Canada's Dalhousie University.

But sometimes you have to sift through more evidence to solve a crime. Here are more unusual strategies to stop kidney stones.

Switch sides. Avoiding kidney stones might be as simple as rolling over. Research by Dr. Marshall L. Stoller of the University of California at San Francisco shows that people who develop kidney stones on one side of the body also sleep on that side. He's not sure why, but theorizes it might have something to do with the change in blood flow to your kidneys caused by the sleeping position.

If you usually sleep on your right side, try sleeping on your left instead, and vice versa. You might get rid of those annoying stones. If you have trouble doing this, you can try the old tennis ball trick, a common way to stop snoring. Sew a tennis ball into the side of your pajamas, so you won't stay in that position. Or use a sleeping wedge to keep you facing the proper way during the night.

Trim the fat. Norman also explored the relationship between dietary fat and kidney stones. In one study, the link was stronger than anticipated – fat had a greater effect on kidney stones than was previously believed. However, in another study, he found no link at all between dietary fat and kidney stones. "There is no association between dietary fat and risk of kidney stone formation in people with a normal gastrointestinal tract," Norman says, adding, "Diet should be one of moderation and variety."

You might not have to worry about kidney stones, but since fat contributes to so many health problems, like heart disease, stroke, diabetes, and cancer, it might be a good idea to limit your dietary fat anyway.

Pass on protein. A French study found that cutting your normal protein intake by about one-third can help protect against kidney stones. People in the study limited meat and fish to three servings a week and didn't have more than 100 grams of milk and cheese a day. Instead, they ate more pasta and rice. To give you an idea of how little 100 grams is, consider this. A cup of skim milk is 245 grams and a 1-ounce slice of mozzarella cheese is 28 grams.

"Protein intake increases urinary uric acid, which can increase stone risk through several mechanisms," Norman explains. The goal is to keep your calories from animal protein at less than 10 percent of your total calories. Nonanimal sources of protein include beans, peas, seeds, and grains.

Go bananas. Getting the recommended dietary allowance (RDA) of potassium might not be good enough to prevent kidney stones. You need more, especially if you eat a lot of salt. A study from Brazil found that, although people ate plenty of potassium-rich foods and their total potassium intake was within recommended levels, they weren't getting enough potassium to combat kidney stones. Potassium helps by increasing the level of citrate in your urine.

Make an effort to eat more potassium-rich foods. These include dried apricots, bananas, tomatoes, oranges, avocados, figs, beans, and baked potatoes.

Tasty ways to 'liquidate' painful stones

Thirsty? If you want to combat kidney stones, you'd better be. Harvard studies show that the people who drink the most fluids have a better chance of avoiding these painful nuisances. In one study, women who drank at least 11 8-ounce beverages a day were 38 percent less likely to develop kidney stones than women who drank less than six. Similar results were found in another study of men. The men who drank the most fluids had a 35 percent lower chance of getting kidney stones than those who drank the least.

But that's not the whole story. What beverage you choose also makes a difference. Here are the best – and worst – beverages to drink if you want to minimize your risk for kidney stones.

- Coffee. A piping hot cup of coffee might be just what you need to wake up and bring down your chances of getting kidney stones by 10 percent. Like alcohol, caffeine waters down your urine and makes you go to the bathroom more often. That gives kidney stones little chance to develop. Oddly, decaf coffee also lowers your risk by 9 to 10 percent. This leads researchers to believe that something other than caffeine is at work.

- Tea. Even though tea was suspected to be high in oxalate, a substance that can contribute to kidney stones, the Harvard studies found that tea lowered men's kidney stone risk by 14 percent and women's risk by 8 percent. That's probably because very little of the harmful oxalate is absorbed by the body. Researchers figure the increased flow of diluted urine caused by the caffeine in tea counteracts the small increase in oxalate.

- Lemonade. This refreshing beverage contains a lot of citric acid, which is a part of citrate. Because citrate stops calcium-based stones from forming, one of the common causes of kidney stones is a lack of citrate in the urine. A University of California at San Francisco study tested lemonade on a small group of people with low levels of urinary citrate. Lemonade more than doubled the amount of citrate in the urine while also cutting down on the calcium. So next time you sip a cool glass of lemonade on a hot day, remember you're also putting kidney stones on ice.

Not all citrus fruits make good kidney stone-fighting drinks. Grapefruit juice actually increases your risk for kidney stones by as much as 44 percent. Researchers aren't sure why, but suspect that grapefruit juice might increase your body's absorption of oxalate from other foods. Another beverage you might want to avoid is apple juice, which increased men's risk for kidney stones by 35 percent but did not affect women's risk.

Wine and beer were actually the most effective beverages in preventing kidney stones in the Harvard studies. Alcohol likely helps fight kidney stones by making you urinate more often and by diluting your urine.

However, alcohol contributes to so many health problems, including liver disease, pancreatitis, high blood pressure, and congestive heart failure, that it's not wise to take up drinking just to battle kidney stones. If you don't drink, don't start. If you do drink, limit your alcohol intake to one or two glasses of wine or beer a day.

Lactose intolerance

The latest buzz on lactose

If you think you're lactose intolerant, think again. Even if you have the nausea, cramps, diarrhea, and bloating that normally come with this condition, you might actually suffer from another problem entirely.

Rule out other causes. Before you take any drastic steps, make sure you really are lactose intolerant. Other sugars besides lactose sometimes cause the same unpleasant reactions.

Your problem could stem from fructose, found naturally in fruits and honey. It's also used in corn syrup to sweeten foods, gums, candies, and sodas. Other culprits include the sugar substitutes sorbitol, mannitol, and xylitol, which are used in sugarless or diet foods, beverages, and gums.

Many people have trouble absorbing these common substances. If you eat too much of these foods, the sugars that aren't absorbed move into the large intestine and cause the same problems as lactose intolerance.

Don't forget about gluten, either. This protein in wheat, rye, barley, and oats gives a lot of people trouble. You could just be sensitive to gluten or have celiac disease, in which case gluten actually damages your intestines. You'd experience weight loss, bloating, gas, weakness, and changes in your bowel habits.

If you have celiac disease, you must completely avoid foods containing gluten. You'll have to read labels carefully since gluten pops up in all sorts of unexpected places – even ice cream. Keep a food diary so you can pinpoint which foods cause which symptoms. This will help your doctor determine your problem.

Beware of hidden lactose. Like gluten, lactose crops up in some unlikely places. If you are lactose intolerant, stay alert.

For example, whey, the watery liquid that's left when milk becomes cheese, is in many processed foods, like crackers. And it contains lactose. So does dry, or powdered, milk. Perhaps most alarming is that about 20 percent of all prescription drugs and 6 percent of all over-the-counter products contain lactose. Make sure you read all food and drug labels very carefully, and ask your pharmacist about any medication you're not sure of.

But even careful attention to labels can't entirely protect you. According to *FDA Consumer* magazine, current labeling guidelines leave some loopholes. Manufacturers can use the term "nondairy" even when the product contains milk byproducts.

And there are more than a dozen ways to include milk protein in the list of ingredients without actually using the word "milk." If you are particularly intolerant, limit your processed foods and avoid anything with unfamiliar ingredients.

Become creative. Don't let lactose intolerance stop you from enjoying food. Try making some substitutions in your recipes. For example, if something calls for dry milk, try using the same amount of water instead. Experiment. You might find some interesting, and tasty, solutions.

It's possible you can dabble in dairy products now and then. While some people, often those of Asian or African descent, are very sensitive and must avoid all lactose, others can eat a small amount. Know your limit, and make sure your menu doesn't go over it.

Macular degeneration

Spectacular ways to keep your eyes healthy

As you stroll through your neighborhood, you may notice the vibrant colors of nature – red, orange, gold, and green. Look for these same colors on your plate at mealtime, and you'll increase your chances of keeping the sights around you in sharp focus.

Eating lots of brightly colored fruits and vegetables can reduce your risk of age-related macular degeneration (AMD), the number one cause of blindness in older people. AMD occurs when the macula, the central part of your retina, breaks down. Nobody knows for sure why this happens, but free radical damage from light exposure is probably a contributing factor.

You won't feel pain with macular degeneration. It just becomes harder to make out fine details as your central vision blurs or distorts. You're considered at risk of developing AMD if you're far-sighted, smoke, have light-colored eyes, spend a lot of time in the sun, or have a family history of AMD or heart disease.

There are two kinds of AMD, wet and dry – both irreversible. Most people have the dry kind, which progresses slowly and generally causes less-serious vision loss. About 10 percent, however, have the wet kind that can cause permanent vision loss within weeks or even days. Although there are some new medications and surgeries for AMD, so far they've had only limited success. The experts say prevention is still the best medicine and a good place to start is with your diet.

Since high blood pressure and heart disease are risk factors, if you cut fat, especially saturated fat, from your diet, you'll be ahead of the game. Then eat lots of dark green leafy vegetables. One research study found that those who ate the most collard greens and spinach had a far lower rate of AMD. Read on to find out more about the nutrients you need to keep your eyes healthy and your vision sharp.

Vitamins and minerals. You know how important teamwork can be in a family or when playing a sport. Vitamins and minerals work together in the same way to help prevent macular degeneration. Healthy eyes have a high concentration of the antioxidant vitamins C and E. They help each other and end up protecting your retinas from free radical damage. Another team player is selenium, a trace mineral that combines with vitamin E to protect your eyes from the dangers of oxidation.

You can get these important team players from the food you eat. Meat, shellfish, fresh vegetables, and unprocessed grains provide plenty of selenium. And you'll absorb lots of vitamins C and E from vegetables and fruits, like apricots, carrots, and red and green peppers. Supplements don't seem to give the same protection, and they certainly don't offer the delicious flavors or other nutrients of these foods.

Carotenoids. Many fruits and vegetables get their bright colors from a group of chemicals called carotenoids. And the antioxidant power of these nutrients can really brighten up your eyesight as well. Two in particular – lutein and zeaxanthin – accumulate in the macula of your eye where they help filter out damaging light rays.

To get lots of lutein, dish up an extra helping of corn and a big serving of those green leafy vegetables. One of the best ways to get zeaxanthin is to add some chopped orange peppers to your green salad. You'll find plenty of both of these carotenoids in zucchini, yellow squash, orange juice, and kiwi fruit. Another good source is egg yolk.

Zinc. You don't need very much zinc, but it's amazing what your body does with just a little. This mineral shows up in every organ, helping with many body processes that keep you healthy. It's especially concentrated in your retinas where it fights free radicals and helps in other ways to protect your eyes from AMD. Researchers have found a relationship between low levels of zinc and a higher risk of AMD.

You probably get plenty of zinc from your diet, but young children, pregnant women, and seniors can sometimes be deficient. Foods that contain zinc include oysters, crab meat, beefsteak, poultry, enriched cereal, and yogurt.

Your body absorbs zinc best from meat, but vegetarians who eat whole-grain breads leavened with yeast shouldn't be deficient in this important mineral.

Some doctors treat macular degeneration with zinc supplements. If you have AMD and think these might help you, be sure to discuss it with your doctor first. There is a real danger of getting too much zinc from supplements.

Fatty fish. To reduce your risk of AMD even more, make fatty fish, like salmon or tuna, a regular part of your weekly menu. The omega-3 fatty acids found in these kinds of fish may protect and restore the cell membranes in your retina.

But eating fish more often isn't necessarily better. Too much omega-3 fatty acids can interfere with your body's ability to use the vitamin E your eyes need.

Wine. Getting important flavonoids from an occasional glass of wine can mean less chance of developing AMD. Pour a glass just once a month, and you'll receive the benefits. Yet, research shows that people who drink beer increase their risk of AMD.

Save your sight with spinach

Spinach may be the best-kept secret in the produce department. It's loaded with nutrients, including many antioxidants. It's rich in carotenoids and is a good source of iron, magnesium, manganese, folate, and vitamins A, C, and K. It's also a dieter's dream.

Just don't think like Popeye and reach for spinach when you've run out of other options. Make this nutritional powerhouse part of your everyday menu to maintain your vision.

The two most common causes of losing your sight in your senior years are macular degeneration, which affects your retina, and cataracts, which affect your lens. Spinach may help ward off both these sight stealers.

Your eye's retina is extremely rich in the carotenoids lutein and zeaxanthin. Experts believe these antioxidants protect your eye from light damage and also support the blood vessels to your retina. Boosting the amount of lutein and zeaxanthin in your body can keep your retina strong and efficient – able to fight off the damage that may cause macular degeneration.

In fact, research found that people who took in more carotenoids decreased their risk of developing age-related macular degeneration by 43 percent. Spinach and collard greens, both containing high amounts of lutein and zeaxanthin, were the foods most closely linked to this protection.

Damage from free radicals may also cause cataracts, a clouding of your lens. But once again, lutein and zeaxanthin come to the rescue. A 10-year study of 36,000 men discovered those who ate the most spinach were protected.

For the best vision defense, eat these leafy greens at least twice a week – more if possible. And if you want to get the most lutein from your spinach, do what Southern cooks have been doing for years – add a little bit of fat, like heart-healthy olive oil. A small amount of fat will increase how much lutein your body can absorb.

Memory loss

Helpful hints to mind your memory

Once upon a time, you could rattle off birthdays, phone numbers, and addresses, keep track of appointments without using a date book, and remember every funny story from your childhood. Now, you're lucky if you remember what you ate for lunch. If your memory batteries seem to be running low, try these tips for recharging them.

Aim for more antioxidants. Many foods contain naturally occurring chemicals called antioxidants that fight damaging free radicals in your body. Beta carotene, which your body converts to vitamin A, is an antioxidant. By protecting your brain cells, beta carotene helps you think, reason, and remember.

Unfortunately, millions of people throughout the world don't get enough vitamin A. Even just 1 milligram (mg) of beta carotene a day makes a big difference. Carrots, sweet potatoes, apricots, tomatoes, broccoli, cantaloupe, and collard greens are all good sources.

Vitamins C and E also fight free radical damage and poor memory. In fact, vitamin E might help ward off Alzheimer's. Look for vitamin C in oranges, grapefruit, broccoli, peppers, cantaloupe, and strawberries. You can find vitamin E in wheat germ, nuts, seeds, and vegetable oils.

Gather memories with herbs. Ginkgo and ginseng both boost memory and concentration. They also fight stress and anxiety and give you energy.

In clinical studies, ginkgo increased blood flow to the brain by 70 percent in seniors. That means more brainpower and better short-term memory. This ancient herb also helps fight signs of dementia, like depression, confusion, absentmindedness, tiredness, dizziness, tinnitus, and headaches. Look for pure ginkgo biloba extract (GBE or GBX). Herbal experts recommend taking 40 mg three times a day. Be patient – it might be a few weeks before you notice results.

To get the benefits of ginseng, chew on ginseng roots or make tea from a small chunk of root. You can also buy a variety of ginseng products, including teas, capsules, extracts, tablets, wine, chewing gum, cola, and candy. Read labels to make sure they contain between 4 and 7 percent ginsenosides, the steroid-like compounds found in the bark or outer layer of the root.

Give your mind a workout. Read, solve a crossword puzzle, take night classes, or find new hobbies. Just keep your mind challenged. Your brain needs to stay in shape to perform at its best. Vary your activities to maximize your brainpower.

Sip, slurp, and swallow. Just because you're confused or show other signs of dementia doesn't mean you have Alzheimer's disease. It might mean you simply need to drink more water. Dehydration causes confusion, disorientation, and other problems. Drink water even if you're not thirsty.

Beef up your B's. Folate, thiamin, B6, and B12 are B vitamins that play important roles in brain function. No wonder people with chronic vitamin-B deficiencies score lower on memory and problem solving tests, while those receiving a boost of B vitamins perform better. A shortage of B vitamins may even lead to Alzheimer's disease. For folate, eat spinach, beets, avocados, asparagus, and other vegetables. Low-fat cheese, fish, and poultry supply you with B12, and potatoes, beans, and watermelon provide B6 and thiamin.

Break those bad habits. Smokers and heavy drinkers already have plenty of health risks. Add memory loss to the list. A recent study of 3,000 elderly men showed that those who smoked throughout their middle years were one-third more likely to have memory loss than men who had never smoked. Even those who once smoked but quit had some memory loss. In addition, alcohol kills brain cells, and drinking heavily (more than two drinks a day) reduces blood flow to the part of the brain that makes memories.

Get your 40 winks. Sleeping is a natural way to boost mind-improving hormones. Not getting enough sleep harms your ability to store information in your long-term memory. Aim for a regular sleep routine – go to bed and wake up at the same time every day.

Start the day off right. Breakfast gives your brain the fuel it needs to start the day. When you wake up, help yourself to a bowl of cereal or a bagel. Studies show children who eat breakfast do better on tests than those who skip this important meal. Other studies suggest something sugary, like sweetened cereals or orange juice, can give your brain a boost.

Check those medications. Your memory loss may not have anything to do with you. It could be a side effect of your prescription drugs. Check with your doctor about trying a different medication.

Lubricate your brain. In an Italian study of nearly 300 seniors, those who ate at least 5 tablespoons of heart-healthy olive oil a day tested best on memory and problem solving skills. It's the monounsaturated fat that enhances your brainpower, but olive oil also has vitamin E and other antioxidants. Whenever possible, use olive oil instead of corn or soybean oils.

Iron out your wrinkled memory. Having trouble concentrating? Don't let a deficiency in an important trace mineral impair your mind. Poor memory could be a sign of iron deficiency, especially if you're pale and feel sad and tired. If you're a vegetarian or regularly take nonsteroidal anti-inflammatory drugs (NSAIDs), you may not be getting enough iron. Even though you find iron mostly in meat, you can also get it from legumes and green leafy veggies.

Safeguard your memories as you age

If you think getting older automatically means your memory goes downhill, think again. A recent study in *The Journal of the American*

Medical Association (JAMA) found that cognitive decline is not a normal part of aging for most people. Seventy percent of the study's elderly subjects showed no significant loss of brain function over a 10-year period.

So don't assume that aging takes away your brain power. You can do a lot to keep your brain sharp for the rest of your life, even if you live past 100.

Avoid atherosclerosis. As you get older, your arteries gradually become less flexible, which could affect blood flow to your brain. If fatty deposits have built up in your arteries, you're even more likely to suffer a loss of brain power. The JAMA study found that people with severe atherosclerosis are at a much higher risk for memory loss.

To keep your brain functioning at its peak for years to come, control your risk factors for atherosclerosis now. A high-fat diet, smoking, and a sedentary lifestyle can make you more susceptible to atherosclerosis. So can high blood pressure, high cholesterol levels, and diabetes. It's important for you to learn more about these conditions so you can avoid them.

Keep moving. You know exercise is good for your body, but did you know it's also good for your mind? Aerobic exercise may be particularly effective. One recent study found that small increases in aerobic fitness improved mental fitness, especially functions that control the ability to plan and organize. You don't have to join an aerobics class, either. Study participants engaged in brisk walking as their aerobic exercise.

And a recent study on mice indicated that exercise may even stimulate the growth of new brain cells, which until recently was not believed to occur in adult mammals.

Break the stress cycle. Cutting stress from your life completely may be an impossible task, but if you value your memories, you should at least try to control your stress.

Research shows that extreme stress causes your hippocampus to shrink. This is the part of your brain most closely involved with memory. A study of Vietnam vets with post-traumatic stress syndrome found that those who spent more time in combat had significantly smaller hippocampi. You may not have the stress level of a soldier in combat, but controlling your anxieties may help you hold onto your pleasant memories a little longer.

Feed your brain. Your brain needs nourishment just like your body. A large study of people over age 60 found memory problems in almost 20 percent of those who skipped meals or did not eat enough. Only 7 percent of those who ate regular meals had poor memories.

Get plenty of vitamin E. The same study found that elderly people with low levels of vitamin E were more likely to have poor memories. Foods high in vitamin E include wheat germ oil (and most plant-based oils), peanuts, and mangoes.

Fight Father Time with prunes

Scientists have wondered what people can do to hold on to the health and vitality of their youth. The latest thinking is that free radical-fighting antioxidants are the key to staying young and avoiding cell damage.

Researchers have measured and studied antioxidants in food at the Jean Mayer USDA Human Nutrition Research Center on Aging at Tufts University in Boston. Of all the foods tested, the prune had the highest Oxygen Radical Absorbance Capacity (ORAC) score. At 5,770 ORACs per 3 1/2-ounce serving, it registered more than twice as many antioxidants as the next highest food, its wrinkled cousin the raisin.

When animals were given foods high in antioxidants, they showed less sign of aging on memory tests. Scientists think antioxidants may be an important key to protecting yourself from diseases of aging and even cancer. In fact, the loss of brain function in certain diseases like Parkinson's and Alzheimer's seems to be from free radical damage.

The USDA's Agricultural Research Service Administrator Floyd P. Horn has seen the future of treating age-related diseases, and it looks a lot like your grandma's vegetable garden.

"If these findings are borne out in further research," he says, "young and middle-aged people may be able to reduce risk of diseases of aging – including senility – simply by adding high-ORAC foods to their diets."

By studying blood samples from different groups of people, the researchers concluded that you can raise the levels of antioxidants in your blood by eating more fruits and vegetables.

For now, they're recommending you eat enough fruits and vegetables to total between 3,000 and 5,000 ORAC units of antioxidants daily. Since most of the foods tested scored in the hundreds, you'd have to eat many servings to reach 3,000.

But chew on this – eating just seven prunes a day can put you well over the 3,000 mark. All the other fruits and vegetables you eat would be extra. Make sure you eat a variety of fruits and vegetables. Each one has different protective nutrients.

Menopause

Natural ways to manage menopause

There are many reasons why you would turn to herbs and nutrients to combat menopause symptoms. Perhaps hormone therapy is simply not right for you, physically or emotionally.

Sit down with your doctor and assess your overall health, your risk for osteoporosis and heart disease, and the pros and cons of aggressive drugs. Then explore alternative therapies. After all, they are the source of many traditional medications.

Cool down with cohosh. If hot flashes and mood swings are bothering you, black cohosh could be just the thing you need. Once called squaw root, Native Americans used this plant for thousands of years to treat female problems.

Today, many doctors in Germany often prescribe black cohosh to treat PMS symptoms, as well as anxiety, mild depression, and sweating in menopausal women. The plant has an estrogen-like effect and reduces levels of a hormone that causes hot flashes. You'll find it in capsules where supplements are sold. Many experts recommend taking 40 milligrams (mg) a day, but not for longer than six months.

Rely on St. John. Hippocrates of ancient Greece recommended the popular herb St. John's wort for menstrual problems. Over two thousand years later, menopausal women still use it to feel better. Best of all, it seems to have very few side effects. Although you may have to stay out of strong sun to avoid a rash, people rarely show allergic reactions.

Be sure the supplement you buy is a reputable brand and contains 0.3 percent hypericin, the active ingredient. The usual dosage is

300 mg, three times daily. Talk to your doctor about using St. John's wort for longer than a few weeks.

Add vitamin A. Most women over age 50 need 700 RE (retinol equivalents) of vitamin A every day. You can get this naturally in the form of beta carotene. Dark green and yellow-orange fruits and vegetables are good sources. During menopause, vitamin A can help counteract dry skin and fight uncomfortable yeast infections. It's also a powerful antioxidant and can help prevent cancer.

Build up your B's. Vitamins B2, B6, and B12 are water-soluble vitamins your body flushes out daily. That means you need to replace them often. They help you turn food into energy; fight migraines, osteoporosis, and depression; and keep your heart healthy. Eat liver, mushrooms, whole grains, bananas, nuts, seeds, eggs, fish, and cauliflower.

Depend on E. Don't let heart disease sneak up on you in middle age as it does for many women. Vitamin E is a major antioxidant that could help keep cholesterol from damaging your arteries. It can also reduce hot flashes and keep your skin soft and younger looking. Add vitamin E to your diet with nuts, seeds, avocados, and canola oil.

Count on calcium. Some health professionals see a connection between low calcium intake and hot flashes. That means a glass of skim milk might keep you feeling cool long after you drink it. In addition, calcium is very important for strong bones. For more calcium, eat yogurt, cheese, spinach, beans, Chinese cabbage, seeds, and almonds.

Study the soy issue. You might want to consider replacing your estrogen with plant sources. Called phytoestrogens, they can give you some of the protective benefits of natural estrogen. Soy-based foods, like soybeans, tofu, miso, and soy nuts, seem to help many women. However, many health experts have concerns. Although some research shows soy improves thinking, helps your heart, and prevents osteoporosis, others suggest it makes your brain age faster.

The latest buzz is the more soy you eat, the greater your risk of developing senility. Talk to your doctor about eating soy during menopause. If you decide to try it, remember this. Because it comes from a bean, you might feel gassy at first, so add it to your diet gradually. And, as in most things in life, moderation is best.

You can find out more about sailing through menopause naturally by consulting a naturopathic physician (ND). These doctors specialize in alternative treatments – no drugs or surgeries. To find an ND near you, go to the Worldwide Directory of Naturopathic Practitioners, Colleges, and Organizations on the Internet at <www.naturopathics.com >. Or contact:

The American Association of Naturopathic Physicians
8201 Greensboro Drive, Suite 300
McLean, VA 22102

(703) 610-9037

Motion sickness

Ease symptoms with anti-nausea nutrients

If you've ever felt the dizzy, unconnected feeling of motion sickness, you know how easily it can ruin a trip. Whether you're traveling by car, boat, or plane, you probably don't care why you're feeling miserable, you just want to feel better.

Motion sickness starts in your ears. That's because they're your body's center of balance. Inside your ears are thousands of tiny nerve endings filled with fluid. The fluid supports tiny pebbles, one in each nerve ending, and when your body moves, the pebbles move with it.

The motion of these pebbles sends messages to your brain, telling it what your body is doing, whether you are sitting, standing, or in motion. When this mechanism is not working right, your brain receives confused or incorrect messages from the nerve centers in your ears, and this confusion can cause nausea.

These mismatched signals can result from an ear infection; ear damage; or from drastic, unusual motion. Sometimes, if your eyes are focused on something moving, like a wave, and your body is moving differently or not at all, like on deck, your brain receives two sets of conflicting messages. Your eyes tell your brain the world is moving, but your ears tell your brain you are standing still.

While it is not known why some people suffer from motion sickness and others don't, it is clear that several factors, including nutritional deficiencies, can lead to ear damage, which can impair the balancing function of your ears.

The following vitamins and minerals can help keep your inner ear in top shape and help fight motion sickness.

Vitamin D and calcium. These nutrients are important to inner ear health. Not only is vitamin D important by itself, a lack of vitamin D can lead to a calcium deficiency. One of the best sources of vitamin D is fortified milk, and it's also a great source of calcium. Other good sources of vitamin D include eggs, green leafy vegetables, and fortified cereals. For a nondairy source of calcium, try some peanuts or broccoli.

Magnesium. A deficiency of this mineral is linked to hearing loss. Squash, potatoes, skim milk, and oatmeal are all good ways to boost your intake of magnesium.

Zinc. This mineral is another important nutrient many older people don't seem to get enough of. Some studies suggest this may contribute to the ear damage and hearing loss that frequently occurs in older people. Zinc is abundant in meats, shellfish, and poultry. You can also get it from legumes, such as black beans, and whole grains. Don't take zinc supplements without checking with your doctor. Zinc supplements can cause serious side effects in high doses.

Why Ginger was everyone's favorite castaway

Ginger has been used for thousands of years to treat everything from constipation to impotence. However, numerous recent studies prove that ginger is an effective remedy for the symptoms of motion sickness. When taken a half hour before traveling, ginger can prevent the nausea that comes from rocking boats or swerving cars.

In one test, powdered ginger was tested directly against Dramamine, an over-the-counter motion sickness drug. The people who took ginger lasted, on average, almost twice as long in a rotating chair as those who took the drug. In fact, half the people treated with ginger did not experience motion sickness at all.

Ginger doesn't affect your inner ear, and it doesn't work on your central nervous system. Rather, it works in your gastrointestinal tract to soothe the vomiting reflex and reduce nausea.

You can buy ginger at any supermarket or health food store. You'll find it in its natural form or as a pill or a powder. A typical capsule, containing 500 mg of ginger, should usually be enough to head off your weak stomach. Some herbal experts recommend taking one or two tablets 30 minutes before your activity, then repeat as symptoms develop.

Candied ginger is a tasty way to enjoy ginger's benefits. This sugary treat can be found at many Oriental markets. A 1-inch square of the crystallized snack equals the amount of ginger in one 500 mg tablet.

If you're still not sure about this natural remedy, try a variation that could very well be in your refrigerator right now. That's right, naturally, not artificially, flavored ginger ale has been used for years to calm hostile stomachs and tame nausea.

What to eat and avoid to fight nausea

What should you eat to help soothe a queasy stomach? Ask 10 motion sickness sufferers, and you'll probably get 10 different answers. Although very little research has been done on home remedies for motion sickness, miracle foods and folk remedies abound. You never know what might work for you.

Pickled okra, anyone? Strange as it may seem, some people swear by pickled okra as a way to fight the motion of the ocean. Dill pickles, olives, and cheese are other pet remedies often used to prevent seasickness. Others suggest sucking on a wedge of lemon to reduce saliva in the mouth and reduce nausea. The most widely recommended food for dealing with the nausea of motion sickness is soda crackers. These plain, dry snacks help get rid of excess saliva and absorb stomach acid that can upset an empty stomach. Soda crackers could be the most tried-and-true of all folk remedies.

Keep your strength up. If you've already gotten sick, it's a good idea to eat something, if you can, to prevent weakness and increased discomfort. Nutrients and electrolytes that you lost during vomiting need to be replaced. Once again, soda crackers can come in handy, since they are bland and absorbent. If you can't eat, try drinking some ginger ale or a cola drink. As a last resort, sucking on some hard candy is better than nothing at all.

Although these remedies haven't been tested in a lab, they have been proven in the field. The best idea, however, is the same as for any allergy or sensitivity. Don't be afraid to experiment a little in order to find out what works – and what doesn't work – for you.

Just say no. While some foods can help ward off motion sickness, there are others you should definitely avoid. In one study, researchers measured motion sickness in pilots and found that the pilots who ate foods high in sodium, such as preserved meats and potato chips, had much higher rates of sickness.

The same was true for high-protein foods, like cheeses and meats, as well as foods high in thiamin, such as pork, eggs, and fish. In addition, foods high in calories also tended to increase the frequency of motion sickness.

In general, avoid strong-smelling, strong-tasting foods. These have a way of filling you up, and they are more likely to trigger a reaction in your sensitive gastrointestinal tract. Instead, try to eat light meals when you know you will be traveling. Reach for bland, low-fat, starchy foods than rich or spicy foods.

Caffeine is an irritant for many people who suffer from motion sickness, and it can bring on bouts of dizziness, especially in people who suffer from Meniere's disease. The same is true for salt. Reducing your intake of these might serve to lessen the uncomfortable effects of motion sickness.

Smoking cigarettes or using other tobacco products increases your risk of motion sickness. Another very common irritant is alcohol, which directly affects your sense of balance. There's no better way to ensure a bout of motion sickness than to start a trip with a drink or a hangover.

Osteoarthritis

At-home plan to stop OA

Osteoarthritis (OA) is the most common form of arthritis. Four out of five adults age 50 or older suffer from one form of OA or another. The "wear and tear" of a long life plays a big part in developing this disease.

Years of moving your joints can rub away your cartilage. This soft tissue normally buffers the end of your bones and prevents them from rubbing together. Without it, your bones scrape together, causing terrible pain. But some scientists also believe an enzyme imbalance in your joints might contribute to the problem. If you have too much of certain enzymes, your cartilage will break down faster than it can rebuild itself.

Although people used to believe it was just a normal part of aging, some experts now think you can prevent this type of arthritis by living a healthy lifestyle. Everyday nutrients appear to be a winning weapon in the battle against osteoarthritis. Although not all experts agree, it's possible the foods you eat could slow and even stop the damage to your joints.

Shedding some pounds if you are overweight might also be a way to halt OA. Those extra pounds add up to more wear and tear on your knees, ankles, hips, back, and other joints that support you.

So it's a good idea to eat foods like fruits, vegetables, and whole grains, which will help you manage your weight. And limit your intake of fatty and sugary foods, while getting your protein from legumes and fish instead of red meats.

Eating a healthy diet can't replace your doctor's advice and treatment, but it can give new hope for a future without painkillers and canes. That's why it's important to evaluate your food choices and make sure you're getting enough of these nutrients in your diet.

Vitamin C. You might think of a bowl of oranges as a toolbox for your joints. Experts say the vitamin C in those juicy treats seems to slow the damage of OA. It might even repair damaged cartilage. The reason behind it is simple – your body needs vitamin C to make collagen, a protein that builds new cartilage and bone.

Besides oranges, eat grapefruit, strawberries, and fresh, uncooked foods, like sweet red peppers and broccoli. Also, make it a practice to sprinkle lemon juice or parsley on cooked foods to replace the vitamin C lost during cooking.

Boron. You're probably not getting your fill of this trace mineral. Most people only get 1 to 2 mg a day. But according to British scientist Dr. Rex E. Newnham, 3 to 10 mg a day could help prevent arthritis. That same amount could also relieve morning stiffness and other arthritis symptoms.

Newnham's research suggests boron is an essential ingredient for bone and joint health. It could also help your body stop calcium loss. Either way, its effects are plain to see. In comparing people who got a lot of boron in their diets to those who didn't, Newnham found that people in boron-rich countries were less likely to develop osteoarthritis.

Snack on noncitrus fruits like apples and pears, a few tablespoons of peanut butter, and a handful of raisins or prunes to reach your joint-saving quota of boron. You might not see results for a month or two, but be patient to reap the benefits of this mineral.

Vitamin D. Research has shown that without enough of this fat-soluble vitamin, you may be more at risk for osteoarthritis of the hip. If you already have OA, vitamin D might slow the condition's progression. Ample amounts of vitamin D can help your body regulate its calcium levels and help regrow new cartilage. Getting your daily dose of "the sunshine vitamin" could be as easy as fishing or golfing on a sunny day. Your body can make this vitamin when enough sunlight hits your skin. But you can still get this essential vitamin if you live in a cloudy part of the world, like New England or Vancouver. Just eat plenty of low-fat dairy products, eggs, and seafood to get your full supply of vitamin D.

Ginger and turmeric. Try these spices and you might be able to cut back on your painkillers. Both contain curcumin, a phytochemical with proven anti-inflammatory powers. It may even work as well as nonsteroidal anti-inflammatory drugs (NSAIDs) like aspirin and ibuprofen, according to the latest research. Brewing ginger tea is a delicious way to add curcumin to your diet. Or toss some fresh ginger or ground turmeric into your next stir-fry. It's a good idea to talk with your doctor first if you have gallbladder trouble or take NSAIDs or blood thinning medication like warfarin.

Water. Making new cartilage for your joints could be as easy as drinking eight 6-ounce glasses of water each day. This pure beverage is a key ingredient in that bone-protecting tissue. To make your daily goal of eight glasses, stick with simple water. Sugary drinks can lead to weight gain, and remember – you want to stress your joints as little as possible.

Ease your pain with this scarlet fruit

Life might not always be a bowl of cherries – but if it were, it might not be quite as painful.

That's because scientists say cherries can relieve pain. Long used as a folk remedy for gout, cherries now carry the clout of scientific evidence.

A recent study by researchers at Michigan State University found that anthocyanins, the same compounds that give cherries their red color, also help squash inflammation. These compounds stop the enzymes that make prostaglandins, hormone-like substances that cause inflammation and pain. Prostaglandins are the bad guys that aggravate conditions like headaches, arthritis, and gout.

Eating cherries every day may help relieve those conditions, says Dr. Muralee Nair, an MSU researcher. "If you have pain from chronic arthritis, and aspirin bothers your stomach, eating a bowl of cherries may reduce that pain," he says.

In fact, laboratory tests showed that 20 tart cherries were at least as effective as other pain-killing remedies, including aspirin, ibuprofen, and other nonsteroidal anti-inflammatory drugs. In some cases, they were much better.

"Cherry compounds are about 10 times more effective than aspirin," Nair affirms.

If you don't feel up to eating a whole bowl of cherries, you can get the same benefit from just a few dried cherries. One dried cherry equals about eight fresh ones.

Recharge your joints with glucosamine

There's good news for you if you're among the growing number of people considering glucosamine sulfate for relief from the pain of OA. Glucosamine, found naturally in the body, gives strength and rigidity to the cartilage that cushions your joints and keeps your bones from rubbing together.

Glucosamine supplements are supposed to help rebuild your damaged cartilage, but most research has not been clear on the benefits of glucosamine in treating osteoarthritis. A new long-term study from Belgium, however, presents convincing evidence glucosamine can bring long-lasting pain relief to your aching knees. In the study, those with OA who took 1,500 mg of glucosamine daily reported less pain and disability. And those good results continued throughout the full three years of the study.

Researchers also found evidence that glucosamine helps prevent wearing away of cartilage in the knees. Those who took placebos, pills that contained no active ingredients, lost space between the bones of their joints during the study. But those taking glucosamine had no significant narrowing of joint space.

You'll need patience if you decide to take glucosamine since it takes about a month to get results and perhaps eight to 12 weeks for the full effect.

Nonsteroidal anti-inflammatory drugs (NSAIDs), such as aspirin and ibuprofen, act faster on OA pain, but they can cause gastrointestinal bleeding and liver damage. Glucosamine doesn't seem to have any serious side effects. And once it kicks in, it's likely to be just as effective as the NSAIDs.

You can buy glucosamine by itself or combined with another supplement, chondroitin, which is also effective in relieving knee pain and improving mobility. Chondroitin is available by itself, too, and appears to have even fewer side effects then glucosamine. But both are made from animal products – glucosamine from clamshells and chondroitin from cow tracheas. Make sure you're aware of possible allergic reactions.

Whether you consider taking glucosamine, chondroitin, or the combined supplements, the Arthritis Foundation offers the following suggestions:

- Don't stop taking your current medications without talking with your doctor. It's also important to discuss the potential benefits and any possible allergic reactions or other problems that might arise from taking these supplements alone or in combination with your other medicines.

- Be sure you actually have OA. These supplements are not recommended for other kinds of arthritis. If you have joint pain and you think it might be caused by OA, see a doctor, preferably a rheumatologist, for an accurate diagnosis.

■ Children and pregnant women should not take glucosamine or chondroitin supplements since the safety and side effects aren't yet clear for these groups.

■ If you have diabetes, consult your doctor about glucosamine. It's an amino sugar, so you may need to have your blood sugar levels tested more often if you take it.

■ Be careful about taking chondroitin if you're on blood thinners, including aspirin. It has a similar molecular makeup to the blood thinner heparin.

The FDA does not regulate dietary supplements, so be sure to buy them from well-known companies. Read the labels carefully, and look for those that give you a total of 1,500 mg of glucosamine. The usual dosage is 500 mg three times a day.

For chondroitin, aim for 1,200 mg total, or 400 mg three times a day. Discuss these supplements with your doctor before you take them. She can help you decide if they're an appropriate treatment for your arthritis.

Tackle arthritis with these 10 tips

Much of life involves learning to cope with challenges and finding out which strategies work for you and which don't. If you have arthritis, here are some ways you can adapt your surroundings to make your challenges easier to meet:

■ To make a pen or pencil easier to grasp, have someone twist a large rubber band around it just below the area where your fingers rest. Or take the plastic center out of a foam hair roller and slide a pencil into the center of the foam. You can also get a pencil grip made of soft rubber where school supplies are sold. A ballpoint pen is easier to use than a felt-tip pen or pencil.

■ Ask someone to help you raise your bed. You won't have to bend over when you make it. Using knitted sheets that stretch will also help you make your bed with ease.

■ To help you tuck in your sheets and blankets, use a wooden pizza paddle.

■ Consider buying a speakerphone to replace your regular telephone so you don't get a stiff or sore neck and shoulder from cradling the receiver for long periods of time.

■ When you're reading, place the book on several pillows in your lap to raise it to a comfortable height. To turn the pages of a book, use the eraser end of a pencil or a rubber fingertip. Blow gently along the edges to separate the pages.

■ To play a game of cards without aching hands, insert the cards into the side of a closed box of aluminum foil or waxed paper. You can also put the bottom of a shoe box into its lid and stand cards in the space between the box and the lid. I

■ n your kitchen, create a lower work space so you can sit while working. Pull out a drawer and place a cookie sheet over the opening. Roll jars and bottles on the counter instead of shaking them. Open a bottle or jar more easily by having someone wind a rubber band around the lid.

■ If you have trouble gripping your car door handle, especially when it's cold or wet, glue a piece of rubber (like the kind that opens jars) to the underside of the door handle.

Make your steering wheel easier to grip by padding it with a foam cover (available in automotive stores). And add extra cushioning to the car seat to keep your back, hips, and legs more comfortable while driving.

■ If you have trouble standing up for a shower, try putting a webbed lawn chair in the shower stall so you can sit while you bathe. It's easier to dry off after a shower by putting on a terry cloth bathrobe. And if you're bathing a baby in a sink or bathtub, wear a soft cotton glove on the supporting hand to keep him from slipping out of your grasp.

■ When you're getting dressed, put the garment on your weaker limb first. When undressing, take the garment off the stronger limb first. Try knee-high or thigh-high hose to eliminate the hassle of putting on pantyhose.

Osteoporosis

How to defend yourself against 2 dangers

If you've got thinning bones, you may have heart disease, too. At least in women, low bone density appears to go hand in hand with hardening of the arteries. So if you're fighting one disease, you might as well fight them both. Follow these proven steps to a healthier heart and beefier bones.

Cash in on calcium-rich foods. If you're over age 50, you need 1,200 milligrams (mg) of calcium every day. Of course, dairy foods are the top sources of this bone-building mineral, but you'd be surprised what other foods can deliver calcium to your plate. Surprisingly, a tablespoon of blackstrap molasses has 172 mg of calcium, while a half cup of collards has 179. Look for other nondairy foods fortified with calcium, like breakfast cereals and orange juice. By increasing your calcium intake to protect your bones, you're also getting a nutrient vital to healthy blood pressure and cholesterol levels, as well as a steady heartbeat.

Pounce on produce. The more fruits and veggies you eat, the stronger your bones. At least that's what some researchers say. A group of men increased bone density and lowered their risk of breaking a hip with every extra vegetable or fruit serving they ate every day. There's a good chance that magnesium and potassium are behind these amazing results. Your body needs these two essential minerals to take advantage of calcium and build bones.

For a healthy heart, it's also important to make potassium and magnesium key ingredients in your daily diet. They are essential for keeping your arteries clear, your heart strong, and your cholesterol and blood pressure low. Avocados, prunes, and dried figs and apricots provide lots of potassium. For marvelous amounts of magnesium, munch on nuts, beans, cereals, bananas, and oranges.

Shake off your taste for salt. In your body, calcium and salt compete in a race to get absorbed. Sometimes extra salt wins and calcium passes right on out. What's more, when you eat too much salt, your kidneys work very hard to flush it out, and they often end up flushing out other important minerals, like calcium, too.

Need another reason to slow down on salt? The connection between a high-salt diet and high blood pressure is well known. Even if salt doesn't affect everyone this way, play it safe for the sake of your heart and bones.

Give up soda. This everyday beverage can be a problem because of its high phosphorus content. Too much phosphorus can interfere with your body's ability to absorb and use calcium. Convenience foods, which are often high in phosphorus and sodium, also leach away the calcium your body needs to build strong bones and control blood pressure.

Fight back with estrogen. Start taking estrogen early and you could cut your risk of hip fracture in half. Estrogen plays a direct role in how well your body builds bone, and it may help with calcium absorption. To get the most benefit from HRT, some experts recommend beginning a program as soon as you notice the first signs of menopause. It's shown to increase hip and spine bone mass by 5 to 10 percent.

Unfortunately, HRT can have troubling side effects – including an increased risk of breast cancer. Meet with your doctor and weigh the upside and the downside before making a decision.

Lose weight without losing bone. Here's the skinny on weight loss – dropping too many pounds could actually lower your bone mass and put you at risk for osteoporosis. Some health professionals think a lower body weight puts less stress on your bones, slowing down the rate they make new cells. Or less weight could mean less fat, cutting down on the amount of estrogen that's available. Either way, this doesn't give you the green light to put on the pounds. Instead, live at a sensible, healthy weight. Talk with your doctor about what weight matches your body frame, sex, and age. Then, achieve it with a balanced diet and exercise.

Working out, don't forget, builds up your bones while burning calories. And many health experts believe an amazing 50 to 70 percent of all heart disease cases stem from obesity. That's enough to make your heart flutter.

Yard work builds strong bones

Working in your yard can do more than give you the most beautiful lawn on the block – it could help give you the strongest bones, too.

Exercise, particularly weight-bearing exercise, helps increase bone density. And a recent study found that gardening may be one of the best activities for building bones.

Researchers found that women who gardened at least once a week had higher bone density than women who did other types of exercise, like aerobics, jogging, swimming, and walking. The only other activity that gave as much protection as gardening was weight training.

What's more, gardening is done outdoors, which exposes women to bone-healthy, vitamin D-boosting sunlight. But perhaps even more importantly, most women enjoy gardening. For any exercise to be effective, it has to be done regularly. And people are more likely to continue an exercise they really enjoy.

So get out there and start digging and weeding. Your bones will appreciate it.

Getting the most from calcium supplements

One of the most common questions Dr. Ann Hunt, Associate Professor of Nursing at Purdue University, gets asked is, "What about supplements?" According to Hunt, not all calcium supplements are created equal, and they work best under specific conditions. Here are some things you should do if you decide to use a supplement.

Check absorption. Most health professionals are concerned with how much calcium actually gets into your bloodstream where it can do your bones some good. This is called absorption. Sometimes the calcium from supplements doesn't make it into your system. The supplement just sits in your stomach, without dissolving.

To test whether or not your body will break down and absorb a calcium supplement, place the tablet in 6 ounces of vinegar or warm water. Then let it sit for about 30 minutes, stirring occasionally. If it's still not completely dissolved after half an hour, it probably won't dissolve in your stomach, either.

Take small doses. Since calcium isn't absorbed very well, Hunt advises taking several small doses throughout the day. "If you take a huge amount of calcium," she says, "only a small percentage is absorbed anyway."

Eat when you supplement. For best absorption, take calcium supplements with food. Hunt explains, "Hydrochloric acid in your stomach helps break down and digest your food. As you get older, your stomach just normally produces less. However, when you eat, your stomach produces extra acid, which then breaks down the calcium." Experts say calcium absorption increases by about 10 percent when taken with food.

Choose wisely. There's a great deal of controversy over which kind of supplement is better – calcium carbonate or calcium citrate. The truth is, Hunt says, they both have pros and cons. "Calcium carbonate is more easily absorbed, but it causes a lot of gastric distress, such as bloating. Calcium citrate doesn't cause as many intestinal problems but less of it is absorbed.

That means you need to take more of the calcium citrate to get your minimum calcium requirements." Read the label for how much of the supplement is absorbable calcium and make a dosage decision you're comfortable with.

Watch your D. Vitamin D plays an important role in how much calcium your bones actually absorb. Studies have proven that low levels of vitamin D go hand-in-hand with weaker, more fragile bones. That's why experts suggest taking vitamin D with your calcium supplements to help reduce your risk of bone fractures.

Hunt says, "You can certainly take too much vitamin D and get into other problems, but 400 to 800 international units (IU) a day is about right."

Your body manufactures vitamin D when exposed to sunshine, but during the winter you are exposed to less sunshine and may experience more bone loss. In addition, sunscreens will block some of your body's absorption of this important vitamin. You don't need to sunbathe in January or give up your sunscreen, just make sure you take in vitamin D from good nutritional sources each day.

Fortified milk is the richest food source of vitamin D. You can also find it in other fortified dairy products and cereals; egg yolks; liver; and fatty fish, like salmon, tuna, and sardines.

Parkinson's disease

Natural help for Parkinson's disease

Parkinson's disease is getting more attention lately because public figures like Muhammad Ali and Michael J. Fox have been diagnosed with the disease.

Parkinson's is a disorder in which your brain cells, or neurons, break down. These neurons produce dopamine, a chemical that helps your brain control your muscle movements. When they die, they no longer make dopamine, and your muscles don't work as well. Parkinson's usually affects people over the age of 50, but it sometimes strikes people in their 20s. It is a little more common in men than in women.

The early symptoms of Parkinson's disease are general and easy to overlook. At first, you may simply feel tired and weak. Then you may notice that your hands tremble while at rest. Your muscles may begin to feel stiff, you may move more slowly, and you may have trouble keeping your balance. You might notice a change in your speech, or your handwriting may become much smaller.

If you think you may have Parkinson's, see your doctor. He can prescribe medicine that will help you. The most common is Levodopa, or L-dopa, which changes to dopamine in your brain. However, L-dopa becomes less effective the longer you use it, so you should try to delay taking this medication as long as possible.

While there isn't a cure for Parkinson's yet, if you're diagnosed with the disease, you can take steps to help control it naturally.

Exercise. If you've always been an active person, keep up your normal activities as long as you can. If you're a more sedentary person, now is a good time to start getting your muscles in better shape. It could help delay some of the stiffness and fatigue that Parkinson's can cause. Aerobic and strengthening exercises are beneficial, but just taking a walk every day will help.

Tai chi is an excellent, gentle form of exercise that may also help improve your balance. Most local recreation centers offer classes in tai chi, as well as other exercise classes. Check with your doctor or therapist for programs that fit your needs.

Watch what you eat. Some people with Parkinson's find that certain foods make their symptoms worse. For example, hot, spicy foods may make movement more difficult. Keep track of what you eat, and whether it seems to have any effect on your symptoms.

■ Protein. Researchers discovered that protein can interfere with the body's absorption of L-dopa. If you are taking L-dopa, limit your protein, and try to get most of it at night, when your medicine doesn't have to be as effective.

■ Fat. Everyone knows too much fat is bad for you, but a recent study found that a diet high in fat may contribute to Parkinson's disease. While more studies need to be done to confirm the findings, it's still a good idea to limit your intake of fat, especially saturated fat. Saturated fat is found in animal products, like meat, egg yolks, milk, cream, butter, and cheese. Several vegetable fats, like coconut oil, palm oil, and hydrogenated vegetable oils, are also high in saturated fat.

■ Fiber. Constipation can be a side effect of Parkinson's, so make sure you get plenty of fiber and drink lots of water. Fruits, veggies, and whole grains are good sources of fiber.

Join a support group. You may have a caring family, but they can't understand what you're going through the way another person with Parkinson's can. Joining a support group may help keep you from feeling alone and depressed, and you may get some helpful advice on how others deal with the disease. Call your local American Parkinson Disease Association to find a support group near you, or call the national headquarters at 800-223-2732.

Try therapy. Different types of therapy are available to people with Parkinson's. Physical therapy may help teach you how to deal with your movement problems and increase your mobility. Some people with Parkinson's have speech difficulties because the muscles in the throat and voice box don't work the way they should.

Speech therapy may help you speak more clearly and make your disease less noticeable. Psychological counseling may help you overcome the depression that often accompanies Parkinson's.

Prostate cancer

Say 'No way!' to prostate cancer

Prostate cancer is the most common form of cancer among men and is second only to lung cancer as the leading cause of cancer deaths for men. It tends to be a slow-growing cancer, but it can sometimes be aggressive and spread quickly. Early stages of prostate cancer may not cause any symptoms so it's important to get regular prostate screenings. The American Urological Society recommends a yearly prostate examination for all men over age 40.

Prostate problems can be just an annoyance, or they can be deadly, prostate cancer kills about 40,000 men a year. And treatments for prostate problems can cause serious side effects. Recent information suggests about 60 percent of men who have prostate cancer surgery are impotent a year and a half later. Preventing prostate problems is obviously your best option, and the right foods can provide some natural help.

Lycopene. Harvard researchers created a stir several years ago when they discovered that eating 10 servings of tomato products weekly could dramatically cut your risk of prostate cancer. Lycopene, a carotenoid that gives tomatoes their brilliant red color, is probably responsible for this protective effect.

Processed tomato products such as tomato sauce and ketchup may be more beneficial than fresh tomatoes. This is probably because chopping and cooking the tomatoes helps break down cell walls, making the lycopene easier for your body to absorb. Other sources of lycopene include watermelon, pink grapefruit, and guava.

Vitamin E. A recent study found that men with the highest blood levels of gamma-tocopherol, a form of vitamin E, were five times less likely to develop prostate cancer.

Gamma-tocopherol appears to work with alpha-tocopherol (another form of vitamin E) and selenium to fight cancer. To get a good balance of both forms of vitamin E, eat a variety of vitamin E-rich foods – seed and vegetable oils, nuts, green leafy vegetables, and whole grains.

Zinc. Pumpkin seeds, which are high in zinc, have been used for centuries as a folk remedy for problematic prostates. Zinc may help shrink an enlarged prostate or reduce the inflammation of chronic prostatitis. Good food sources of zinc include oysters and other shellfish, chicken, beans, and whole grains.

Vitamin D. This "sunshine vitamin" may be useful in preventing or treating prostate cancer. However, vitamin D can also be toxic in large doses, so don't use supplements without a doctor's guidance. Instead, eat foods rich in vitamin D, such as dairy foods or fortified cereals, and get out and soak up some sun. Your body can make its own vitamin D from the sunlight on your skin.

Soy and green tea. China has the lowest rate of prostate cancer in the world, and Japanese men are also less likely to develop the disease. It could be that something in the Asian diet helps prevent prostate cancer, and research points to two possibilities – soy and green tea.

Researchers at Loma Linda University found that Seventh-day Adventist men who drank soy milk at least once a day were 70 percent less likely to develop prostate cancer. An earlier study on Japanese men living in Hawaii found those who ate tofu (another soy product) were less likely to develop the disease.

Asians also drink lots of green tea, which may protect against several types of cancer. Green tea contains antioxidants called polyphenols that may be responsible for this beverage's cancer-protective effect.

A recent study suggests a combination of these two Asian staples could be the secret. Scientists found that the polyphenol in green tea did not fight prostate cancer cells in the laboratory by itself. But when combined with genistein, a substance found in soy, the solution halted the growth of prostate cancer cells.

One possible drawback to soy is that it may make your brain age faster, new research claims.

Garlic. This favorite of Italian cooks contains more than just a strong flavor and odor. It may contain strong cancer protection as well. Garlic is loaded with antioxidants and other substances that help boost your immune system and protect against cancer.

Cruciferous vegetables. Broccoli, cauliflower, and brussels sprouts can help you put the squeeze on prostate cancer. Eat just three servings of these cruciferous veggies every week, and you could cut your risk of prostate cancer in half.

Simple steps to a healthier prostate

Prostate cancer affects mostly older men, but it's never too early – or too late – to start a prevention program.

Move it. Exercise may help prevent prostate cancer. Researchers studying almost 30,000 men found that those who were active in their jobs were less likely to develop prostate cancer. If your job requires you to sit behind a desk, don't worry. Leisure time activities also lowered the risk of developing the disease. And you don't have to spend a lot of time or money on exercise equipment. Walking was the activity associated with the greatest reduction in prostate cancer risk.

Lose it. If you're overweight, you're more likely to get prostate cancer, particularly if you gain weight after age 50. One study found that men with a body mass index (BMI) greater than 29 have an 80 percent greater risk of developing prostate cancer than men with a BMI of less than 23. To calculate your BMI, divide your weight in pounds by your height in inches squared and multiply that number by 703.

Cut the fat. Probably the best way to keep your BMI under control is to limit your intake of fat, another risk factor for prostate cancer. Men with the highest fat intake have a 79 percent increased risk of advanced prostate cancer than those with the lowest intake. Try to limit your fat intake to no more than 30 percent of your total calories and reduce your intake of saturated fat to 10 percent or less of your total calories.

Beat it with beta carotene. If you eat lots of brightly colored vegetables and fruits, which are rich in beta carotene, you may be protecting yourself from prostate cancer. A recent study found that men who had the lowest blood levels of beta carotene were 45 percent more likely to develop prostate cancer than men with the highest beta carotene levels. You could be giving yourself a double dose of protection if you eat tomatoes, apricots, and watermelon because they contain both beta carotene and lycopene. Other foods high in beta carotene include carrots, sweet potatoes, pumpkin, spinach, and mangoes.

Skip the smokes. Smoking affects more than just your lungs. It also increases your risk of prostate cancer. One study found that men who smoked 20 cigarettes daily were 2.9 times as likely to develop prostate cancer as men who didn't smoke.

Psoriasis

Self-help made easy

If you want something done right, do it yourself. That seems to be the philosophy of many people with psoriasis. According to the National Psoriasis Foundation (NPF), self-treatment is becoming more popular for people with this skin condition.

You can choose from a variety of alternative remedies ranging from acupuncture to magnets. However, there's little scientific evidence that any of these therapies work. To help make your choice of treatments easier, here are some of the more effective and proven psoriasis self-help strategies.

Hit the beach. This sounds too fun to be therapy, but it's true. Spending some time in the sun and water – a strategy called "climatotherapy" – offers relief to many people with psoriasis. In fact, according to the NPF, 80 percent of those who get regular exposure to the sun show improvement. It's the sun's ultraviolet light that helps clear up your skin.

If you're nowhere near a beach, that's OK. Dr. Steven R. Feldman, a professor of dermatology and pathology at Wake Forest University School of Medicine, recommends an easy solution.

"Of the alternative treatments, the most effective is tanning beds since we know how good ultraviolet light is for psoriasis," Feldman says. "Sunny beach vacations are also outstanding."

Not to mention more fun. The most popular location for psoriasis treatment is the Dead Sea, which offers plenty of sunlight and special water. But traveling halfway around the world might not be the most practical approach.

Don't worry – you can get the benefit of "climatotherapy" at the Jersey shore or any beach near you. Just make sure you sunbathe safely, because too much exposure to the sun can cause skin cancer. Ask your dermatologist about any precautions you should take, such as using sunscreen and avoiding the sun at its peak hours of 10 a.m. to 2 p.m. And enjoy your day in the sun.

Chill out. Stress doesn't only aggravate you – it also aggravates your psoriasis. One good way to keep your psoriasis in check is to keep your stress levels under control.

Studies have shown that hypnosis and relaxation tapes help conventional treatments work better. But anything that helps the mind relax comes in handy. Try stress management techniques such as yoga, tai chi, or meditation. Exercise often cuts down on stress, too. However you do it, relax. It will only make things better.

Go fish. Many supplements claim to fight psoriasis. One that actually works is fish oil. In several clinical trials, fish oil supplements improved the symptoms of psoriasis, including scales, redness, and itching. As a bonus, fish oil also helps boost your mood, improve your memory, and defend against heart attacks and strokes. Another supplement possibly worth trying is evening primrose oil, which helped relieve other skin disorders in a number of studies.

The fatty acids in these supplements protect your skin and fight inflammation, which might have something to do with psoriasis. Just talk to your doctor before taking any supplements.

Rub it in. To treat psoriasis, you need to moisturize your skin. A wide range of topical products – those you apply to your skin – might do the trick. Aloe vera helped treat psoriasis in one study, and other natural over-the-counter moisturizing products could be effective. Bath products that contain oats soothe the skin, while products containing capsaicin helped clear up scaly skin, redness, and itching in some studies. One of the oldest remedies for psoriasis is coal tar, which you can get with or without a prescription. You should probably use it under a doctor's supervision, though.

Feldman says that a combination of a strong cortisone-type medication and an ointment called Dovonex, a substance similar to vitamin D, is the best way to clear psoriasis for those with only a few spots. Ask your doctor about these medications.

"In most cases, it's probably a good idea to see a dermatologist to confirm the diagnosis and to establish a treatment plan," Feldman says. He also says it's important to quit smoking, stop excessive drinking, eat a healthy diet, and exercise regularly.

"Even if these don't help the psoriasis, they are still a good idea," he notes. "Especially the alcohol part, because alcohol can damage the liver, and some of the best medicines for psoriasis can't be used in people with damaged livers."

Raynaud's phenomenon

Hot tips to beat cold hands and feet

Building a snowman, snow skiing, or taking a walk on a clear, cold night are activities that make winter delightful. If you have Raynaud's phenomenon (RP), however, just getting cold can turn into an extended bout with pain. Any exposure to frigid temperatures can bring a stinging and numbness to your hands and feet.

"Even something as simple as filling glasses with ice for a family dinner becomes a real problem for me," says 23-year-old Jennifer, who was diagnosed with Raynaud's five years ago. "After grabbing just a few ice cubes, my hands turn white, then a bluish color, then red. My hands feel numb, then the pain starts."

This extreme sensitivity to cold affects about 10 percent of the population, usually women between the ages of 15 and 50. Raynaud's may strike out of the blue or stem from an underlying condition such as atherosclerosis, lupus, or rheumatoid arthritis. If you work with vibrating machinery, play the piano frequently, or have carpal tunnel syndrome, you're even more at risk.

Oddly enough, it's not just the cold that provokes a painful reaction – emotional stress can do it as well. Prevention is your best weapon in fighting this condition. Follow these tips to lessen your chances of suffering painful fingers and toes.

Bundle up. Medical studies in Great Britain have shown that body temperatures in Raynaud's sufferers drop faster than normal. It also takes them longer to get warm again. That's why it's important to protect yourself from cold at all times. Wear a warm coat, hat, gloves, and boots when you are outside in cold weather. Inside, protect yourself from cold drafts by snuggling in a warm blanket or quilt and wearing socks and shoes or slippers all the time.

Wear gloves in the house. Protect your hands whenever you take a package of frozen food from the freezer or fruit from the vegetable drawer. Keep a pair of clean winter gloves in the kitchen, along with potholders and towels you can fold around cold items while you take out the contents.

Jennifer is always careful to wrap several layers of paper towels around a glass of cold water or a chilled soft drink before picking it up. Insulated drink holders made of Styrofoam are also helpful.

Pamper your pinkies. Keep your hands clean and dry, and try to keep them safe from cuts, scrapes, and bruises. Don't treat them roughly. If you develop any sores on your hands that don't heal, see your doctor.

Turn up the heat with pepper. Spicy cayenne pepper has a pain-relieving and warming effect on your skin. Sprinkle a little into your socks or gloves before you put them on to keep your hands and feet warmer. But first make sure you have no cuts or scrapes on your skin. Wash your hands when you take off your gloves, and be careful not to touch your eyes or nose.

Cut out caffeine. This common drug affects your circulation and can have a negative effect on Raynaud's phenomenon. This includes the caffeine in coffee, tea, chocolate, and colas, and many cold and cough remedies that contain decongestants.

Give ginkgo a go. Ginkgo is an ancient herbal remedy for improving your circulation. It may help your blood vessels stay open to improve blood flow in your fingers and toes. You can buy ginkgo as a food supplement in pill form in your local health food store or drugstore.

Keep your environment smoke-free. If you smoke, give it up. If your friends and family smoke, ask them not to do it around you. Breathing in cigarette smoke takes much-needed oxygen from your body and narrows your blood vessels, making the symptoms of RP even worse.

Check out "helpful" hormones. If you take hormone replacement therapy and have developed RP, there may be a connection. A recent medical study found that women taking estrogen were much more likely to develop Raynaud's phenomenon than those who weren't taking it, or those taking estrogen plus progesterone. If you take estrogen by itself, ask your doctor to change your hormone prescription to help you avoid the symptoms of RP.

Condition yourself. Fight Raynaud's naturally with a technique developed by Army scientists. People in this study held their hands in a bucket of warm water while standing in the freezing cold. They did this for 10 minutes, three times a day, every other day, for a total of 18 days.

At the end of the treatment, the people with Raynaud's had trained the blood vessels in their hands to stay open even when their bodies felt cold. The effects of this particular treatment lasted as long as two to three years.

Try biofeedback. This is another type of conditioning exercise in which your mind trains your body to keep the blood vessels in your hands and feet open when they should be. You can learn to "think" your fingers and toes warm. Check with your doctor to find someone who can teach you this technique.

Smooth out your stress. Stress can make RP worse, even when you are not cold. When you can learn to relax and deal better with your stress, your symptoms of Raynaud's phenomenon may get better, too.

Avoid the causes. Jennifer recommends making choices that won't put you in a painful situation in the first place. "Don't sit down on a cold desk in a classroom or put your hands on a cold doorknob without something between you and the metal," she says. "If you've been out in the cold weather and want to wash your hands when you come inside, don't use either hot or cold water – it will really hurt. Lukewarm is what you want to use."

Your best plan is to stay out of cold environments that you know will bother you, and give these natural remedies a try. Your hands and feet will thank you for it.

Rheumatoid arthritis

Find arthritis relief — on your plate

Your body literally turns on itself when you have rheumatoid arthritis (RA). That's why this devastating condition is called an autoimmune illness. White blood cells, which normally hunt harmful bacteria and viruses in your blood, seem to invade and attack the soft tissues of your joints. Experts aren't sure why the white blood cells go haywire, but they know the symptoms – swollen and throbbing joints.

Like osteoarthritis, RA can lead to permanent damage to your bones, cartilage, and other joint parts. In time, it can even hurt internal organs, like your heart and lungs.

RA tends to attack matching joints at the same time - both knees or both elbows, for example, or your hand's small joints. The best way to prevent the disease from going that far is by getting treatment early. The sooner you begin therapy, the less the condition will disfigure your joints.

Rheumatologists – doctors specializing in arthritis – usually prescribe nonsteroidal anti-inflammatory drugs (NSAIDs) or other strong medications. These can quiet your RA, but they can cause side effects. Relief, however, could be as painless as eating a healthy, balanced diet.

"Certainly," says Dr. David S. Pisetsky, author of *The Duke University Medical Center Book of Arthritis*, "a patient with rheumatoid arthritis who may not be eating well would benefit from a nutritious and well-balanced diet."

Eating high-fiber, low-fat foods will also help you manage your weight, and keeping the pounds off leads to better bone health.

Remember – extra ounces equals added stress to your joints. As Pisetsky states, "Rheumatologists believe that body weight does influence arthritis."

The right foods, together with regular exercise, could make it easier for your body to fight RA. That makes them the perfect complement to your doctor's treatment plan.

Omega-3. According to the Arthritis Foundation, eating fish at least two or three times a week can soothe your stiff, achy joints. You can thank the omega-3, or linolenic, fatty acids. Omega-3 appears to relieve the symptoms of RA so well that some people can cut back on NSAIDs. Stick with cold-water, fatty fish, like salmon, mackerel, albacore tuna, and herring, for the biggest boost. Between seafood suppers, try cooking with canola oil and making salad dressings with flaxseed oil.

Cut back on omega-6, or linoleic, fatty acids, too. While omega-3 reduces the number of enzymes in your body that promote inflammation, omega-6 encourages your body to make more. This is a tug-of-war you want omega-3 to win. To help it win, limit your intake of foods rich in omega-6, such as meats, processed and fast foods, and vegetable oils, like safflower, corn, and soybean.

Olive oil. This fragrant oil turned up the big winner in a recent study from Greece. The researchers surveyed the eating habits of over 300 people in search of foods that can benefit people suffering with RA. Of over 100 types of food, olive oil came out the winner.

The monounsaturated fatty acids in olive oil appeared to work like omega-3 fatty acids by helping to reduce joint swelling at the source. The oil's antioxidants could play some role, too.

Try to work olive oil into your diet almost every day. The more you use, the better. In the study, the people who consumed the least olive oil had a two and a half times greater risk of getting RA than the top olive oil eaters, who averaged three tablespoons more a day.

Antioxidants. Speaking of free radical fighters, exciting new research suggests all antioxidants might relieve, or even prevent, RA. Rheumatoid sufferers tend to be overloaded with free radicals and low on antioxidants. This imbalance leads experts to believe free radicals have a hand in causing joint damage. Eating foods rich in antioxidants could help give the edge back to the good guys, the antioxidants.

There are a few leaders in the antioxidant army – selenium, vitamin E, and resveratrol. In a recent study from Sweden, low selenium levels appeared to increase a person's risk for getting a certain kind of RA. Some experts think raising your selenium intake might even help to reduce your swelling and pain. Low vitamin E levels, on the other hand, raised the risk for all types of RA.

Boost your selenium levels with seafood, mushrooms, dairy, and whole wheat. Rich sources of vitamin E include fortified cereals, vegetable oils, peanuts, and fish.

Resveratrol mainly comes from grapes. Many researchers think it inhibits inflammation, making it a weapon against RA, heart disease, and cancer.

Pumpkin seed oil. You can profit simultaneously from the powers of antioxidants and fatty acids when you cook with pumpkin seed oil. Sometimes called "green gold," this unusual oil contains omega-3 fatty acids, as well as selenium, vitamin E, beta carotene, and other antioxidants called polyphenols.

When you put all of these ingredients together, you get a potent anti-inflammatory remedy. You can cook with it or use it to make your favorite salad dressing. Chefs prize "green gold" because of its unique nutty taste. If you have trouble finding this oil in your grocery store, you can order it through the mail.

Ginger and turmeric. You can ease the inflammation and ache of your next flare-up with a pot of ginger tea or a heaping plate of curry. Turmeric, the leading spice in curry, and ginger both contain curcumin, an antioxidant with pain-fighting powers. In laboratory studies, curcumin appeared to be as potent as NSAIDs, like ibuprofen. The Arthritis Foundation even lists turmeric and ginger as alternative therapies for RA.

Water. Soothing your fiery joints could be as easy as drinking six 8-ounce glasses of water each day. Water lubricates and cushions your joints. But stay away from sugary drinks. They can lead to weight gain, which could make your arthritis worse.

Creative ways to cope with RA

Coping with the pain and exhaustion of rheumatoid arthritis (RA) can be overwhelming – even with prescription medicine. Fortunately, strong medicine isn't your only resource. Many people find relief with alternative remedies. Try these drug-free ways of dealing with RA.

Use that old-time religion. When 35 people with RA kept diaries for a study, researchers learned spirituality can be a key to coping with pain. The people who had daily spiritual experiences – such as being moved by the beauty of creation – were in better moods and had much less joint pain.

These people were also more likely to have a support group to help them when things got rough. Don't let the stress of RA keep you from tuning in to your spiritual side. Stay involved with a group of like-minded people, and your body could profit along with your spirit.

Intensify exercise. You're probably tempted to baby your joints after an RA flare, but experts say you should do just the opposite. In a recent study, people hospitalized for RA were put on a program of muscle strengthening exercises five times a week and bicycle conditioning three times a week in addition to their usual range-of-motion exercises. Another group simply did the range-of-motion exercises. After 24 weeks, the super exercisers had much better muscle strength and were functioning better physically. Ask your doctor about cranking up your exercise program. You may be capable of more than you think.

Keep moving. Have you been skipping your workouts because you'll just have to quit when your RA flares? Keep up the workouts in between, experts say, and you'll do better in the long run. Researchers found that people who backed off on exercise after they had a flare-up felt more upset about their disease and more limited by it as time went on. Stay tough mentally, and don't let RA rob you of any activities without a fight. Even though you have to rest your joints during a flare, get back into action as soon as you're able.

If you need direction and motivation, ask your doctor about physical therapy. In a recent study, people with moderate to severe RA had physical therapists come to their homes for six weeks to teach them about exercise. Another group with similar symptoms did nothing different. After 12 weeks, the group that received physical therapy had fewer tender joints, less morning stiffness, and better grip strength. A follow-up study done a year later revealed that the results were long lasting.

Indulge in a massage. Who wouldn't enjoy a soothing rubdown? It loosens tight muscles and helps you relax – two things you need when you have RA. If you don't have someone at home who can give you a massage, ask your doctor to recommend a professional masseuse. For a special treat, visit a day spa that offers massage. You'll feel pampered and renewed by the time you leave. Just be careful of joints that are painful or inflamed, since massage can make them worse.

Get needled. Acupuncture, which has been around for thousands of years, requires a trained professional to place sterile needles in various parts of your body. Usually the acupuncturist leaves them in for about 20 minutes. Acupressure is similar, but it's done with pressure, not needles. Although the jury is still out on whether or not these practices work, many people claim they have gotten long-lasting relief. If you'd like to try something different, check with your doctor first, then find a licensed acupuncturist or acupressurist. With a little luck, you might even be able to find a medical doctor who performs this service.

Help yourself with herbs. Although using herbal supplements for RA is still controversial, some have been used for centuries with good results.

- Bromelain and boswellia. Scott Zashin, one of the best medical doctors in the country, according to the authors of *Best Doctors in America*, uses conventional and alternative therapies in his practice in Texas. For his RA patients, he sometimes recommends bromelain and boswellia. He says they may reduce inflammation. Bromelain is an enzyme that occurs naturally in pineapple. You can buy bromelain extract in capsules at health food stores and herb shops. The usual dosage is 400 to 600 mg three times a day. Boswellia, also known as frankincense, is used in India as a traditional remedy for rheumatic inflammation. It can slow down inflammation and increase blood supply to your joints. The usual dosage is 150 mg of the extract three times a day.

- Tripterygium. This plant, used in China to treat autoimmune diseases, is also known as "thunder god vine." Studies show it works by partially blocking inflammation. In a 12-week study, people with RA and their doctors said they saw a significant improvement in the participants taking tripterygium compared with a sugar pill.

Rosacea

Proven ways to reduce flare-ups

Legendary comedian W.C. Fields had rosacea, but this condition is
no laughing matter. Rosacea often strikes in your 30s and 40s, but
it may be just as common – and more severe – after age 50.
Women and people with fair complexions get rosacea more often,
but it can affect anyone. It also attacks men and women differently.
Signs of rosacea normally show up on women's cheeks and chins,
while the nose, like that of Fields, becomes the target area for men.

Although rosacea has no cure, you can take steps to manage this
chronic disease. Make a plan for living with rosacea.

Find your triggers. First, you have to discover what sparks your
rosacea flare-ups. Triggers can vary from cold or hot weather to
spicy foods, alcohol, or hot baths. In short, anything that makes
your face flush is a potential trigger. One person with rosacea
might get flare-ups from salsa, while another can eat salsa but
flushes from drinking wine. Therefore, you don't have to give up
everything – just the things that aggravate your rosacea. Keeping a
diary to track your flare-ups might help. Then, once you've determined your personal triggers, make some lifestyle changes to cope
with rosacea.

Modify your diet. What you eat and drink has a big impact on
your rosacea. Besides spicy foods and alcohol, other common culprits include liver, yogurt, cheese, soy sauce, vinegar, sour cream,
citrus fruits, chocolate, vanilla, eggplant, spinach, avocados, hot
chocolate, coffee, and tea.

"Diet seems very important," says Dr. Joel Bamford, a dermatologist at St. Mary's-Duluth Health System in Minnesota. "A lot of our

patients who had rosacea associated theirs with dairy products. You probably don't want to eat a lot of hot liquids or foods. The temperature of food makes them flush. It's a normal thing; it's just more obvious for people with rosacea."

Partly because of Fields' trademark bulbous nose and constant references to drinking, rosacea is often incorrectly linked to alcoholism. In reality, teetotalers can suffer from it just as much. But alcohol does aggravate the condition for many people.

If you do have one too many drinks – or too much chocolate or whatever else triggers your rosacea – and have a flushing episode, Bamford suggests chewing on ice chips for relief.

Protect your skin. It's important to take care of your face. When washing your face, stay away from harsh, grainy soaps and rough washcloths. Rinse with lukewarm water and gently blot your face dry with a soft towel.

Once your face is dry, apply your medication. Then, once that is absorbed, you can put on some camouflaging make-up. Green-tinted foundation helps some people offset the red. Both men and women can use some type of make-up to cover their red spots.

Make sure to use sunscreen, even on overcast days. If it irritates your face, try a brand made for children. These are usually gentler. Don't go outside in the heat between 10 a.m. and 2 p.m., when the sun is at its strongest. Wear a scarf or ski mask in the winter to protect your face from the cold and wind.

Handle your emotions. A survey of 700 people with rosacea by the National Rosacea Society found that for 91 percent of them, emotional stress led to flare-ups. Most common kinds of stress included anxiety, anger, frustration, worry, and embarrassment.

"People call attention to your appearance, so that's embarrassing, and a reason for being more flushed," Bamford says. "And stress can make one flush and contribute to the appearance of rosacea."

Family, jobs, finances, health, relationships, and social pressure caused the most stress. The good news is 83 percent of those surveyed who tried stress management said it helped keep rosacea flare-ups in check.

Bamford suggests deciding if the problem is stress-related first, then coming up with a strategy to deal with the situation. One option, of course, is to avoid what's causing the stress. Another is to talk to a friend, minister, or even a psychologist.

"There's also biofeedback, meditation, tai chi," Bamford adds, noting that each person must figure out what works best for them. "It's such a personal thing, what you do about stress."

Exercise is a great way to work out stress, but don't overdo it. Sometimes during heavy exercise, you become too flushed and bring on a flare-up. Explore different relaxation techniques to see what works for you. You'll stop seeing red – literally.

Sinusitis

Secrets to soothing irritable sinuses

What medical condition makes life tougher than even heart disease or back pain? Would you believe sinusitis? A recent study found that people who suffer from chronic sinus problems experience more pain and less pleasure in their daily activities than people with these and many other chronic conditions.

Your sinuses are air-filled pockets located above and behind your eyes and nose. When the mucus from your sinuses doesn't drain properly from these pockets, it builds up and can become infected. Since you can feel stuffed up at any time, how can you tell the difference between a head cold and a serious sinus condition?

The U.S. Department of Health and Human Services offers this advice: When your sinus discomfort interferes with your life, causes you to miss work or take frequent naps, or is the source of regular colds, infections, or earaches, it is time to see a doctor.

One simple way to see if your sinus problem is serious is to take the jump test, a technique that Dr. Basil Rodansky, the test's inventor, swears by. Simply jump up and down or skip rope for a few minutes, and observe the results. If this causes severe sinus pain, says Rodansky, you probably have acute sinusitis and should consult your doctor.

Avoiding known irritants and allergens can help prevent mild sinus problems. When they do come up, knowing how to handle them can make your life a lot more pleasant.

Sleep soundly. Research shows that not getting enough sleep can make your sinus problems more painful and longer-lasting. Too much sleep, however, can have the same effect. Try to sleep with your head slightly raised to help your sinuses drain at night, or if one side is stuffier than the other, sleep with that side tilted down.

Run for it. For many people, mild to vigorous exercise opens up nasal passages and clears their breathing. Others find it makes their clogged sinuses worse. You should be exercising anyway, so why not give this solution a shot and see if it helps?

Care for your air. Even clean air can irritate sensitive sinuses, especially in winter months when it is particularly dry. Use a humidifier in your home to put moisture back into the air and make it easier to breathe. It keeps your sinuses from drying out.

Go soak your head. Some people get relief by placing warm, water-soaked towels directly over their sinuses, holding their face over a steaming sink, or simply breathing in the steam from a cup of hot water. For an extra boost, consider adding pine oil, eucalyptus, or menthol to the water.

Visit the druggist. Natural solutions are best, but sometimes an over-the-counter decongestant is good for some quick relief. Try to use a decongestant that has only one active ingredient, so there will be fewer side effects, and it will be easier to stop using.

Never use a decongestant for more than three days. Longer than that, and you risk developing a dependency that can cause a "rebound effect." When that happens, the symptoms come back worse after you stop taking the medicine.

Steer clear of blockers. One type of medication you should avoid is antihistamines. These medicines basically dry up your sinuses and cause your mucus to thicken up, which may provide temporary relief but does not solve the real problem. In fact, stopping the regular flow of mucus through your sinuses can actually make the problems worse.

Rinse out your nose. It may sound uncomfortable, but many find relief through nasal rinses you can make right at home. Simply mix a quarter teaspoon of ordinary table salt with 7 ounces of warm water. With a bulb syringe, squirt the solution into your nose and let it soothe and rinse your sinuses.

You can also use a device called a Neti Pot, a spouted container designed to pour water into your nose.

After mixing the salt and water in the container, tilt your head sideways over the sink and pour the solution into one nostril, letting it flow out the other, then repeat with the other nostril.

After 30 seconds or so, use a tissue or your fingers to blow out whatever solution remains in your sinuses. Check your local health food store for the Neti Pot or a similar product.

Rinsing your nose daily may help you avoid colds as well as sinus problems. In a study at Pennsylvania State University, researchers showed that using a daily saline rinse significantly reduced the number of colds among college students.

Try natural relief. There are probably as many opinions out there on natural remedies as there are sinusitis sufferers.

- Some swear by acupressure, in which you apply a few seconds of direct pressure to certain sensitive spots on your face, such as the inner edges of your eyebrows, the sides of your nose, and the bones below and around your eyes.

- Light massage, especially to the area over your sinuses and the muscle between your thumb and forefinger, has been known to bring some relief.

- If all else fails, try crying. Releasing pent-up emotion may also relieve the pressure in your sinuses.

The trick is to find what works best for you, and stick with it. If home remedies fail, and you continue to get worse, make sure you see your doctor before the infection causes lasting damage.

Expert advice for sinus problems

Dr. Robert S. Ivker, author of the book *Sinus Survival*, has been treating people with sinus problems for over 30 years.

He believes the right diet can help heal your sinuses by protecting and healing mucous membranes, strengthening your immune system, and reducing the growth of yeast.

He discusses additional ways to fight sinusitis on his Web site at <www.sinussurvival.com>.

Strive for vitamins and minerals. Delicious, colorful fruits and vegetables, like apricots, cantaloupe, strawberries, red and green peppers, kale, parsley, and broccoli, get high praise from Ivker. They contain lots of vitamin C, which, he says, fends off colds, allergies, and sinus infections.

You also need vitamin A to keep your mucous membranes healthy. If you eat carrots, sweet potatoes, cantaloupe, mangoes, and winter squash, you'll get lots of beta carotene, which your body converts to vitamin A.

Zinc, found in beef liver, dark turkey meat, and black beans, helps change beta carotene to vitamin A. It also helps build up your immunity and reduces the risk of respiratory infections that can lead to colds.

Ivker recommends vitamin E, too, for preventing allergies and sinusitis. And its power, he says, is doubled when you get selenium with it. Whole grains grown in the rich soil of the United States and Canada provide both these nutrients.

Drink more water. Keeping your mucous membranes moist will increase your resistance to infection and allow your sinuses to drain more easily. So drink lots of water – even more than the recommended six 8-ounce glasses a day. For adults who aren't very active, Ivker suggests half an ounce of water per pound of body weight. If you get a lot of exercise, increase the amount to two-thirds an ounce per pound.

For example, if you weigh 130 pounds, you need between eight and 13 8-ounce glasses a day. You can drink less if you eat a lot of fresh fruits and vegetables.

For variety, Ivker suggests herbal teas, natural fruit juices diluted 50 percent with water, or thin soups. Choose products low in salt and without added sugar. Avoid coffee, regular tea, and cola. "Caffeine is a diuretic that can contribute to dehydration and increased mucus production," says Ivker.

Ditch problem foods. You may think of milk, sweets, and alcoholic beverages as comfort foods, but if you are battling sinusitis, they may be adding to your discomfort.

"The change I recommend most," says Ivker, "is to avoid milk and dairy products. The protein in milk tends to increase and thicken mucus secretions." In addition, shun sugar and alcohol, especially if you think a fungal infection may be causing your sinus woes.

"The foods that most strengthen the immune system," explains Ivker, "are also highly beneficial to those whose sinus condition is caused by nasal allergies; these are garlic, onions, citrus fruits, and horseradish."

Skin cancer

Simple steps to protect your skin

Skin cancer shows up most often in people over 50, but it begins when you are much younger. Each time you expose yourself unprotected to the sun, you raise your risk of developing skin cancer – and millions of people are doing just that every day.

The good news is that skin cancer is usually curable if diagnosed early enough. "The difference between life and death is a quarter of an inch," says Dr. Perry Robins, president of the National Skin Cancer Foundation. "If you catch it early, nobody need die."

That's why the two keys to fighting skin cancer are prevention and early detection.

Begin with sun safety. The biggest enemy your skin has is the sun. Ultraviolet rays damage skin cells and can cause them to grow uncontrollably. Protecting your skin from the sun should be your number one priority.

■ Avoid getting too much sun even during the winter and on cloudy days. Be especially careful between 10 a.m. to 3 p.m. when the sun is strongest. If you must be in the sun during this time, wear long sleeves, a hat, and sunglasses.

■ Sunscreen is your next best defense against skin cancer. Choose a waterproof product with sun protection factor (SPF) of 15 or higher, and reapply it often.

■ Use strong sunblock on vulnerable areas like your nose, ears, and lips. In fact, applying lipstick twice a day will cut your risk of developing lip cancer in half. Men need to remember their lips, too. There are several colorless lip balms available that contain sunscreen.

Aim for early detection. Nearly all skin cancers can be cured if found early enough. Your doctor can even remove most growths right in the office. Have her give your entire body a thorough inspection once a year, especially if you are light-skinned. Between professional exams, get in the habit of checking yourself – from head to toe – once a month.

■ Be sure to look at both sides of your hands and at your lower and upper arms.

■ Undress completely and stand in front of a full-length mirror. Look at your whole body, front and back. Raise your arms so you can check under them. Use a hand mirror for any back parts you can't see.

■ Use the hand mirror to examine your scalp, ears, and the back of your neck. To make it easier, part your hair or use a blow dryer for a closer look.

■ Check out the backs of your legs and the bottoms of your feet with the mirror. Look between your toes, too.

What you are looking for is anything new, like a change in a mole or new growths. Be on the lookout for any mole with the ABCDs listed below. They could be the deadliest form of skin cancer – malignant melanoma.

■ A for asymmetry. This means that one side of a mole doesn't match the other.

■ B for border. The border of most moles is smooth. A mole with edges that are irregular, ragged, or blurred could be a warning sign of skin cancer.

■ C for color. A mole that is a mixture of several colors, including blue, red, tan, black, white, or brown could be a red flag signalling melanoma.

■ D for diameter. If a mole is larger than a pencil eraser, have it checked out by your doctor – it could be cancer.

Other types of skin cancer include basal and squamous cell carcinomas. They may look like a pearly bump or a red, scaly, sharply outlined patch. You may think flat moles or patches are harmless, but that's not necessarily true, so talk to your doctor about any new or different skin growths you find.

Get the 'skin'ny on sunscreen

Wearing sunscreen – incorrectly – could put you at risk for melanoma, the deadliest type of skin cancer. If you don't choose the right sunscreen or apply it properly, your skin is in as much danger as if you weren't wearing sunscreen at all.

The whole reason for sunscreen is to protect you from the sun's two types of scorching rays – ultraviolet A (UVA) and ultraviolet B (UVB). Both suppress your immune system and can cause skin cancer. Most sunscreens only block UVB rays, so, for protection from UVA rays, buy sunscreens labeled as "broad spectrum."

Make sunscreen a part of your daily routine, like brushing your teeth or combing your hair. And learn the where, when, and how of good sun sense.

Know your SPF. According to the American Academy of Dermatology (AAD), the Sun Protection Factor, or SPF, is a number that refers to the product's ability to block out the sun's burning rays.

It is figured by comparing the amount of time it takes to burn protected skin, to the amount of time it takes to burn unprotected skin. For instance, if you sunburn without sunscreen in 10 minutes, it would take 150 minutes to burn if you were wearing a sunscreen with SPF 15.

Sunscreen products range from SPF 2 to SPF 60. However, most dermatologists believe an SPF of less than 4 is not really even a sunscreen and anything over 30 offers very little added benefit. The AAD recommends an SPF of at least 15 for everyone, but go for higher protection if you:

- have a light complexion.
- have ever had skin cancer in the past.
- have a family member who had skin cancer.

If you have a serious illness or are on medication, talk with your doctor before spending any length of time in the sun.

Don't skimp. One of the biggest mistakes you can make, experts say, is not putting enough sunscreen on. To get the coverage you need, the average adult should use about one ounce of sunscreen – that's the amount it takes to fill a shot glass.

Plan ahead. It takes 20 to 30 minutes for sunscreen to soak into your skin. So, slather on the lotion well before going outside. This will also give it time to dry so it won't rub off on your clothes or your car seat.

Watch the clock. While a good sunscreen is critical for skin protection, many people believe a high SPF sunscreen means it's safe to stay in the sun longer. This probably explains why people who use a high factor sunscreen still get sunburned. Whatever your SPF choice, experts suggest you keep sun exposure to small doses and reapply sunscreen every two hours.

Rinse and repeat. Going to the beach or pool means extra sunburn risk. Most swimmers will get burned despite the fact they use sunscreen. Even waterproof sunscreens come off after swimming and toweling dry. Play it safe and apply more when you come out of the water.

Don't bug out. Let's say you're bothered by bugs AND the sun. An insect repellent containing DEET will fend off the creepy-crawlies, but it will make your sunscreen a third less effective. On the other hand, a product containing both sunscreen and insect repellent seems to hold off the sun, but not the bugs. You choose which is more important for your outing and take extra precautions, if necessary.

Keep an eye on the index. The National Weather Service and the Environmental Protection Agency (EPA) together developed a scale – from 0 to 10 – to let people know how much UV radiation reaches the Earth at any given time. It's called a UV Index. Use it to decide how much sun protection you'll need for the day.

UV Index Number	UV Radiation Exposure
0-2	minimal
3-4	low
5-6	moderate
7-9	high
10+	very high

You can find the UV Index with your newspaper's weather map, or on the local television or radio daily forecast. Also, look on the EPA's Internet site at <www.epa.gov/sunwise/uvindex.html>.

Stash It everywhere. Keep a bottle of sunscreen in all sorts of places, like your car, pocketbook, picnic basket, or golf bag. Leaving sunscreen out in the heat won't affect how it works.

Be a good role model. Teach your children and grandchildren a valuable lesson. Put your sunscreen on in front of them, and they'll follow your lead to healthy skin.

Put men on alert. It's a scientific fact. Men use sunscreen less often than women and are less careful about how they put it on. That means, men, you're more likely to get a sunburn – and more likely to get melanoma after 40. That's a high price to pay for a little carelessness.

Go for the shade. The best way to avoid burning is to stay out of the sun. Find cover under a tree, a beach umbrella, or a wide-brimmed hat. Wear loose-fitting pants and long-sleeved shirts to protect your arms and legs.

Be especially careful from 10 a.m. until 4 p.m. when the sun is strongest. And remember, just because it's cloudy doesn't mean it's safe. About 80 percent of ultraviolet rays can pass through the clouds and cause skin damage.

Skip the reflection. Sand and water can reflect up to 85 percent of the ultraviolet rays. That makes the beach one big magnifying glass, and it gives you one more good reason to cover up and slap on sunscreen.

Fake a tan. If you want that attractive summer glow without the risk of cancer, wrinkles, and freckles, experiment with one of the new sunless tanning lotions on the market. These actually stain your skin without harming it. Your "tan" will fade in a week or so, but remember, you'll still need to apply sunscreen.

Count your way to cancer protection

Want to figure out your chances of getting skin cancer? Try counting the number of moles you have on your body. Experts say it's a fairly reliable indicator of how likely you are to develop skin cancer. By adulthood, the average person has 15 to 20 moles. If you have more than that, you have a greater risk of developing this disease.

When checking for moles, it is very important to recognize the difference between these types of spots and freckles or age spots. Moles first appear as flat, dark-brown spots, but they eventually rise and become rounded, sometimes turning light brown or pink.

Liver spots or age spots are larger, flat, brown patches that usually appear after age 55, especially on the face and hands.

Freckles are small, flat, brown spots that usually come out after you've been in the sun. You have fewer freckles during the winter, so that may be the best time to count your moles.

Stroke

Take small steps to slash your risk

According to the American Stroke Association, someone in America has a stroke every 45 seconds. And strokes kill 160,000 people each year. Understanding strokes and how to avoid them may keep you from being added to the statistics.

When you have a stroke, the blood supply to your brain is cut off, either by a blockage of blood flow or by a blood vessel that ruptures and bleeds. When the blood supply to your brain is cut off, depriving it of oxygen, brain cells die.

A stroke that is caused by a blockage is called an ischemic stroke. Ischemic strokes can be caused by a blood clot that forms in your brain or neck (thrombosis), by a blood clot that forms elsewhere in your body and moves to your brain or neck (embolism), or by a narrowing of an artery that won't allow blood through (stenosis).

A stroke that is caused by bleeding into the brain or the area surrounding the brain is called a hemorrhagic stroke. These strokes are more often fatal than ischemic strokes. They are sometimes caused by a ruptured aneurysm – a weakened spot in an artery that bulges outward.

Just the thought of a stroke can be frightening, but you needn't feel helpless. There are things you can do to cut your risk.

Kick the habit. Smoking contributes to a buildup of fatty substances that can block the main artery supplying blood to your brain. This type of blockage is the leading cause of stroke in the United States. If that doesn't convince you, consider these facts:

■ nicotine in cigarettes raises blood pressure

- carbon monoxide in cigarettes reduces the amount of oxygen your blood carries to your brain

- smoking makes your blood thicker and more likely to clot

Kicking the habit isn't easy, but when you consider what smoking is doing to your body, it's worth the effort. Your doctor can recommend programs or medications that make quitting easier.

Get in motion. Regular exercise can reduce your risk of stroke substantially because it helps keep your blood pressure under control. Researchers at Yale University found that men who walked over a mile a day cut their risk of stroke in half.

Drink more milk. High blood pressure often goes hand-in-hand with stroke. Since calcium helps control blood pressure, experts wondered if it would also reduce the risk of stroke. Researchers looked at information gathered for 22 years from several thousand men. The risk of stroke was quite different among the men who took calcium pills and those who ate a lot of dairy products.

Men who drank more than 16 ounces of milk a day were half as likely to suffer a stroke as those who didn't drink milk. Those who got their calcium from nondairy sources, such as supplements, had no stroke advantage.

Another study found that women who had a higher calcium intake, whether it was from food or supplements, were less likely to suffer a stroke.

These studies suggest getting plenty of calcium, particularly from dairy products, may help you avoid a stroke.

Eat cruciferous, citrus, and leafy greens. Eating at least five servings of fruits and vegetables a day may lower your stroke risk. A recent study found that the risk of ischemic stroke was 31 percent lower in people who ate more than five servings of fruits and vegetables a day, compared with people who ate fewer than three servings a day. Cruciferous vegetables, like broccoli, cabbage, and cauliflower; green leafy vegetables; and citrus fruits and juices seem to provide the most protection.

Buy into B vitamins. Studies have shown that B vitamins can help lower your risk of suffering a heart attack or stroke by controlling homocysteine levels. This substance, a by-product of protein metabolism, can damage and narrow your arteries.

Taking B vitamins after a stroke may even help heal the damage. In a recent study, researchers divided 50 stroke survivors into two groups. One group took a vitamin supplement containing 1 milligram (mg) of vitamin B12, 100 mg of vitamin B6, and 5 mg of folic acid. The other group took a vitamin supplement without the B vitamins. After three months, the people who were taking the vitamin supplements with the B vitamins had lower levels of homocysteine and thrombomodulin, a chemical indicator of damage to the blood vessels.

Another study found that even among young women, high homocysteine levels were associated with a higher risk of stroke. In the study on women ages 15 to 44, those with the highest levels of homocysteine had double the risk of stroke compared with women having lower levels.

Get plenty of potassium. If you want to lower your risk of stroke, make sure you get enough potassium in your diet. A recent study found that men who had the highest potassium intake were 38 percent less likely to have a stroke than men with the lowest intake of potassium. Good food sources include bananas, dried apricots, avocados, figs, beans, and cantaloupe.

Stop stroke hook, line, and sinker

A fish a day could make stroke go away – almost.

Say you eat fish at least five times a week. You've just cut your risk of suffering a stroke in half. That's a whale of a finding. These promising numbers come out of a recent study published in the

Journal of the American Medical Association. During the course of 14 years, researchers from the Harvard Medical School and the University of Miami School of Medicine followed the eating habits of almost 80,000 women. They came to the conclusion the more fish they ate, the better chance they had of living stroke-free.

Men can net the same benefits. If you eat about an ounce or more of fish per day, you'll have half the risk of stroke as men who reel in less fish. It takes just two delicious filets a week to meet this quota. In fact, just two servings of fish each week will also bolster your body against heart attack, diabetes, depression, and cancer.

The heroes behind these true-to-life fish tales are compounds you probably have heard about before – omega-3 fatty acids that keep blood clots from forming. With names like eicosapentaenoic acid (EPA) and docosahexaenoic acid (DHA), it's easier to eat omega-3 fatty acids than spell them. The best way to do that is by choosing cold-water, fatty fish like anchovies, bluefish, herring, mackerel, mullet, salmon, sardines, sturgeon, trout, tuna, and whitefish.

Actually, some experts believe fish oil is such a powerful anti-clot compound that too much could be dangerous, increasing your risk of hemorrhagic stroke – when blood vessels in your brain rupture and cause internal bleeding.

You don't really have to worry about this, however. Eating like an Eskimo once in a while, according to the Harvard-Miami researchers, does not appear to put you at greater risk for hemorrhagic strokes. For real danger, you would have to eat fish at least three times every day – getting around 3 grams of omega-3 fatty acids.

If any amount of fish is too much for you, you can get omega-3 fatty acids from landlubber foods. Try flaxseed, walnuts, and dark leafy greens like collard, spinach, arugula, Swiss chard, and kale.

By including these foods in your regular diet, you'll not only protect your brain from stroke, but also guard against arthritis, skin problems, and immune system imbalances.

Watch out for hidden triggers

What do snoring, drinking beer, and taking aspirin or decongestants have in common? Believe it or not, they may all give you a stroke. Knowing about such unexpected, hidden risks as these – and how to deal with them – just might save your life.

Check your breathing. Your spouse's snoring may be so bad that you're ready to sleep in another room. But wait. Before you leave him on his own, check to make sure he's not suffering from a potentially deadly sleep disorder. Consistent snoring can be a sign of sleep apnea, a dangerous condition that could put him at severe risk for a massive stroke.

During an attack of sleep apnea, you stop breathing momentarily. The struggle to breathe causes your blood pressure to shoot up, damaging the carotid arteries that carry blood to the brain. Putting these critical arteries in jeopardy puts you at terrible risk for stroke.

Sleep apnea is seen most often in overweight people and can be treated. If you suspect you or a loved one may suffer from sleep apnea, see your doctor or visit a sleep clinic as soon as possible.

Ditch your decongestant. If you use an over-the-counter medicine to clear up that stuffy nose, you might want to reconsider. Research shows that long-term use of a common decongestant called pseudoephedrine may trigger a stroke, especially in those who suffer from migraines or Raynaud's phenomenon. If you are using this medicine and have one or more other stroke risk factors, ask your doctor about alternatives.

Cut your beer intake. Too much alcohol opens the door to many health problems, but heavy beer drinkers may have more to worry about when it comes to stroke risk.

A study at the Innsbruck University Clinic in Austria found that people who drink more than four beers a day tend to have more fatty buildup in the arteries leading to their brains. This type of blockage can cause an ischemic stroke. The study found that heavy beer drinking was an even bigger risk factor for stroke than smoking 20 cigarettes or more a day.

Evaluate aspirin's pros and cons. For years, you've heeded the advice to take aspirin to help control your risk of heart disease. While this may be sound advice for protecting your heart, doctors have now found it might not be so good for your brain.

Researchers at Johns Hopkins and Tulane universities analyzed 16 studies involving subjects who had suffered hemorrhagic strokes. This type of stroke occurs when a weakened artery bursts in your brain. They found that although aspirin makes you less likely to have a heart attack or ischemic stroke, it may increase your risk of having a hemorrhagic stroke.

The researchers concluded that the benefits of aspirin therapy for your heart probably outweigh the danger it poses in stroke risk. But this may not be true for all people. If you are at particular risk for hemorrhagic stroke, be sure to discuss this with your doctor before starting an aspirin-a-day routine.

Stroke symptoms? Call 911!

When it comes to stroke, timing is everything. A delay in treatment could mean the difference between life and death, or between complete recovery and living with paralysis.

A drug called tissue plasminogen activator or tPA (trade name: Activase) dissolves blood clots that cause ischemic strokes, making recovery more likely. For tPA to be effective, it must be given within three hours of the stroke.

It's important to know the warning signs of stroke:

◆ Numbness or weakness of an arm or leg, especially on one side of the body

- Sudden confusion or trouble speaking
- Dizziness
- Loss of balance or coordination
- Blurred or double vision
- Sudden, severe unexplained headache

If you think you are having a stroke, call for emergency medical help immediately.

Guard against food-drug interactions

Blood thinners could save your life – or end it. This type of medication protects many people from life-threatening blood clots. But certain foods and herbs interact with blood thinners like warfarin, putting you in danger of a particular type of life-threatening stroke.

If you have a family history of hemorrhagic stroke – when a blood vessel in your brain ruptures – and if you take warfarin, you must be especially careful to avoid these deadly interactions. In addition, if you have high blood pressure, you're more at risk of a hemorrhagic stroke since the walls of your blood vessels are weak and more likely to burst.

Learn what can interact with warfarin, and talk to your doctor about your risk.

Vitamin K. You need this vitamin for your blood to clot properly, but when paired with warfarin, it can spell trouble. A single large intake of vitamin K can block warfarin and cause dangerous blood clots. Don't cut out all foods rich in K – just don't go to extremes. Eat foods like broccoli, Brussels sprouts, kale, parsley, spinach, egg yolks, liver, and vegetable oils on a regular schedule. For instance, eat three servings of broccoli each week – not six servings one week and none the next. Also, avoid taking large doses of vitamin K supplements without the approval of your doctor.

Garlic. The same compounds that make this spice a superstar heart healer could also make it dangerous for people taking blood thinners. Garlic naturally stops your blood from clotting. Taking two blood thinners at once – your medication and garlic – could lead to uncontrollable bleeding.

That spells hemorrhagic stroke if it occurs in your brain. To avoid this, experts warn against taking standardized garlic extract. They also suggest eating no more than one clove of garlic a day.

Ginkgo. In a few isolated cases, mixing warfarin and ginkgo has led to dangerous internal bleeding. That's because ginkgo, like garlic, keeps your blood cells from clumping and forming clots. So, before taking gingko, talk to a doctor or pharmacist.

Vitamin E. This vitamin, by itself, is a blood thinner. Combine it with warfarin and you run the risk of thinning your blood too much. But you can play it safe by avoiding large doses of vitamin E, over 400 International Units (IU) a day, while you're on warfarin. Eat E-rich foods such as avocados, nuts, seeds, and wheat germ in moderation.

Papaya. A compound in papaya, called papain, could also make warfarin's effects stronger. So, ask your doctor before you eat papaya or take products with papain in them.

Alcohol. Alcohol can cause your body to process blood thinners more rapidly. An occasional drink shouldn't be a problem, but don't dramatically change your drinking habits while you're on warfarin. And always drink in moderation.

Warfarin reacts with a wide variety of over-the-counter and prescription medications. Be careful with aspirin, acetaminophen, antibiotics, and certain drugs for high cholesterol and ulcers. Ask your doctor how much – if any – is safe to take.

A delicious nutty side dish may save your life

Try some tabbouleh instead of potatoes and you'll add more than just variety to your diet. Research says eating whole grains like bulgur cuts your risk of stroke, cancer, type 2 diabetes, and heart disease.

Stops stroke. In one study of more than 75,000 women, those who ate the highest amount of whole grains cut their risk of an ischemic stroke almost in half.

Curtails cancer. Whether it's the fiber, antioxidants, or phytoestrogens that do the trick, bulgur battles digestive system cancers, like colon cancer, and hormone-related cancers, such as breast and prostate cancer.

Holds up heart disease. Whole grains are good for your heart because they help control your weight, lower your blood pressure, and reduce bad LDL cholesterol levels while keeping your good HDL cholesterol steady.

Drop-kicks diabetes. It's no secret, people who eat whole grain foods on a regular basis are less likely to develop diabetes. And since whole grain products tend to have a low glycemic index, bulgur is a good food to include in your diet if you're diabetic.

Tinnitus

Tame tinnitus with these tactics

Tinnitus and rest don't go together very well. Just try sleeping with a constant ringing, clicking, hissing, roaring, or whistling sound in your ears. That's bad enough, but when you don't get enough rest, your levels of stress and tension increase – and stress and tension can make your tinnitus worse. It's enough to drive you crazy.

"There's no question that stress and tension do exacerbate tinnitus," says Jack Vernon, one of the foremost experts on the condition. "So you want to avoid that if at all possible."

While there's no cure for tinnitus, there are plenty of management strategies. Read on to discover how you can take steps to deal with tinnitus, handle stress, and get the rest you need.

Run a background check. "I tell patients two conditions to religiously avoid," says Vernon, former director of the Oregon Hearing Research Center. "The first is loud sounds because we know they can permanently increase tinnitus. The second is total quiet. Always have some background sound playing."

This approach, called "masking," covers up the sound of the tinnitus, which becomes much more noticeable in complete silence. Masking devices you wear in your ear, like hearing aids, are available. You can also try music; tapes of environmental sounds; or other soothing, distracting noises.

The Oregon Hearing Research Center sells Moses-Lang compact discs, which contain seven 10-minute bands of noise, each at an increasingly higher pitch. You can listen to the CD, find the noise that best blocks out your tinnitus, and set your bedside CD player on repeat so you hear that noise all night long. An even simpler solution is to adjust your bedside FM radio between stations so you get static. This often masks tinnitus.

And yet, not everyone responds to masking. "I tell them to do the faucet test," Vernon says. "Go to the kitchen sink and turn the water on full force. If the sound of running water makes it impossible, or nearly so, to hear the tinnitus, it's highly likely that masking will work for them."

The following treatments are similar to masking.

- Hearing aids. Sometimes simply treating your hearing loss helps mask your tinnitus. That's because you suddenly hear the creaks, whirs, and other background sounds of everyday life that you've been missing. These noises effectively block out the tinnitus. You can even find a combination hearing aid/masking device if neither one helps by itself.

- Tinnitus Retraining Therapy (TRT). This technique combines low-level, steady background sounds with one-on-one counseling until you grow unaware of tinnitus and eventually no longer need to wear devices in your ears. Although quite effective, TRT can take up to two years to work. "I think most people are interested in more rapid relief," Vernon says.

Attack anxiety. If masking doesn't work, Vernon recommends the anti-anxiety drug Xanax, whose generic name is alprazolam. In a study conducted at Oregon Health Sciences University, 76 percent of those treated with alprazolam experienced relief from tinnitus. The decibel (dB) level of their tinnitus also decreased.

"When loudness was actually measured, it went from a 7.5 dB average to a 2.3 dB average," Vernon says. "If people can get down to 2.3 dB, there will be dancing in the streets."

Of course, Xanax will also help your anxiety and stress. Ask your doctor about this prescription medication. You might also want to try sleep medications if the nighttime is especially difficult for you.

If you'd rather not rely on drugs, why not try these other stress-busting strategies.

- Relaxation therapy and visualization. By using focused breathing and positive imagery, you learn to relax. That means less stress and, possibly, less severe tinnitus.

- Biofeedback. This helps you monitor and control your body's reaction to stress. Often used in conjunction with relaxation therapy, biofeedback uses your own nervous system as an ally in the fight to stay healthy.

- Yoga or meditation. These methods of relaxation and focusing help some people with tinnitus.

- Exercise. Sometimes activity can be distracting. While you're jogging or playing tennis, you won't be focusing on the tinnitus.

Join the club. You're not in this alone. Look for a tinnitus support group where you can learn from others and share your experiences with the condition. Many people find this helpful.

It might also be a good idea to join the American Tinnitus Association. This organization sponsors research for tinnitus. The more support it gets, the more research it can sponsor – and the closer they will get to a cure. Plus, becoming a member will help keep you up to date on the latest breakthroughs.

Remember, you don't have to use just one treatment option. Mix and match to find what works for you – but do something.

TMJ

How to grind a bad habit to a halt

Did you know that your teeth, on average, can bite down with a force of 162 pounds per square inch (psi)? If that sounds like a lot, imagine a biting force of 975 psi – that's the record for teeth grinding. It's no wonder that this condition, called bruxism, can cause serious dental damage.

Bruxism can also lead to TMJ (temporomandibular joint disorder). The temporomandibular joints on each side of your head connect your upper and lower jaws to each other and to your skull. They allow your jaws to open and close, rotate, and move back and forth. When these joints become damaged, it can cause pain in your ear, teeth, jaw, neck, and head.

Some of the other symptoms of TMJ disorder are a clicking or popping sound when you open your mouth or chew, pain when you yawn, and the inability to open your mouth widely. Although there are several possible causes of TMJ, it seems bruxism accounts for many cases.

Besides running the risk of developing TMJ, people with serious bruxism will have teeth that appear flat on the surface, because they've worn them down. You can even wear the enamel off your teeth, exposing the dentin, which is the inside part of your tooth. Your teeth then become very sensitive, particularly to temperature extremes of hot and cold.

All the painful problems bruxism can lead to makes it painfully obvious that you need to find a way to stop the grinding.

Reduce stress. The best way to stop grinding your teeth is to get rid of the stress that's causing it, but for most people, stress is an inescapable fact of life. However, finding effective ways of dealing with it may help. Since most teeth grinding occurs at night, a relaxing bedtime ritual like taking a warm bath or reading may help. For severe stress, however, counseling may be best.

Change your sleeping position. The position you sleep in can make a difference. The best way to sleep is on your back with pillows or rolled-up towels under your knees and neck. This allows your lower jaw to relax. If you can't sleep on your back, sleep on your side with supports under your head, shoulder, and arm. Sleeping on your stomach is not recommended.

Have someone wake you. Often, you don't even realize you're grinding your teeth in your sleep until your spouse complains that the noise is keeping him awake. If this is the case, ask your spouse to wake you whenever he notices you grinding away. This may help break the cycle and condition you to stop before you have to be awakened.

Get a mouthguard. Your dentist can fit you with a mouthguard, similar to the ones worn by boxers, only smaller. This device may or may not stop you from grinding your teeth, but it will help protect your teeth from more severe damage.

Eat soft foods. Bruxism causes your jaw muscles to become tired and overworked. Give them a break by eating soft foods and staying away from hard, chewy foods like bagels.

Avoid chewing gum. You may think chewing gum helps relieve the stress that makes you grind your teeth, but it uses the same overworked jaw muscles. You're better off without it.

Use your imagination. Visual imagery and relaxation techniques may help reduce stress and loosen up that tight jaw. Think about relaxing your jaws with your lips closed and your teeth apart. Try to do this about 50 times a day, until you're comfortable doing it. Then visualize sleeping with your jaw in that position, and soon you may be free from the nightly grind.

Toothache

Preventing cavities in 'grown-up' teeth

Less than one out of three seniors has dentures today. Only 30 years ago, more than two out of three seniors had false teeth. These statistics sound like a dental miracle, but if you're a senior with your natural teeth, think about this. More than 95 percent of seniors have receding gum lines, and this leaves their roots open to attack by decay-causing bacteria. No wonder tooth decay is three times as likely in seniors as it is in children.

How can this be? Teeth you've had your entire lifetime can wear out just like any other part of your body. There are also other reasons why your teeth are under attack, and all of them are under your control.

Brush like you were 20 again. Doing a good job brushing and flossing can be tricky if you have arthritis or other health problems. Yet, without good oral hygiene, you're at the mercy of millions of bacteria, and they have no mercy.

One simple solution is to buy an electric toothbrush. Just point this modern marvel at your teeth, and let it do all the work. You can also redesign your traditional toothbrush to make it easier to grip. Widen the handle by attaching a bicycle handle grip, a sponge, or a rubber ball. With a wooden ruler or a tongue depressor, you can also make your toothbrush handle longer. Do both by wrapping adhesive tape around your toothbrush until the handle is the perfect length and width. For flossing ease, make your string into a loop or buy a special floss holder.

Ask your doctor about side effects. Medications that cause dry mouth can put you at risk for tooth decay. These include decongestants, antihistamines, painkillers, and diuretics. Saliva not only lubricates your mouth, it washes away food that normally gets stuck between your teeth. More importantly, it dilutes the bacterial acid that causes cavities. That's why a parched mouth spells trouble for your teeth.

To get your juices flowing again, talk with your doctor about switching medications. In some cases, she might be able to prescribe another medicine that won't sap your saliva. For quick relief, enjoy a piece of sugar-free candy or gum. They encourage your salivary glands to produce more saliva.

Don't turn your back on fluoride. Drinking bottled or purified water might be putting your mouth in danger. That's because these sources of water are short on fluoride, the mineral that's famous for guarding teeth. Most towns and cities add fluoride to their water supplies, but if you're drinking bottled or purified water, you're missing out.

If you don't want to give up your bottled water, consider this surprising source of fluoride — carbonated soft drinks. Most brands, according to recent research, contain almost as much fluoride as most tap water. But remember, the sugar could undo any benefit the fluoride has. If you enjoy an occasional soft drink, stick with the sugar-free varieties.

Leave your fears behind. Avoiding the dentist can be downright dangerous, leading to tooth loss and gum disease.

Dentistry has come a long way. Gone are the days of painful drilling with a foot-pedaled drill. Dentists today have the talent and the technology to make your next visit comfortably pain-free. If you're unhappy with your dentist, find one that helps you feel comfortable. Don't let bad memories from your childhood prevent you from having a healthy mouth.

Snack wisely. Experts say when you eat is as important as what you eat. Eating during scheduled meal times is much better for your teeth than nibbling on snacks throughout the day. Each snack you eat leaves your teeth open to attack from bacteria for at least 20 minutes. Meals cause less damage because you have more saliva in your mouth during a full meal. If you have to snack, stick with these nutritious choices – veggies, cheese, plain yogurt, or a piece of fruit.

Listen up, denture wearers. Don't think you can avoid taking care of your mouth just because you wear dentures. According to experts, you're still at risk for mouth cancer, gum disease, and mouth sores.

Visit your dentist at least once a year. She can check your mouth for signs of trouble and make sure your dentures fit well.

Ulcers

The best way to heal an ulcer

Ulcer sufferers used to have a hard life. They were trapped in strict diets, warned to avoid stress like the plague, and often blamed for their predicament. Fortunately, health experts now know differently. Being stressed out or eating spicy or acidic foods doesn't cause ulcers, but they can aggravate an ulcer you already have.

Most ulcers are caused by *Helicobacter pylori*, cork-shaped bacteria that burrow into your stomach's protective lining. This attack allows digestive acids to burn through the lining and cause the ulcer, or sore, in your stomach or small intestine.

Kill the *H. pylori* and, in most cases, you'll heal the ulcer. Antibiotics do the trick for most people.

So visit your doctor if you suspect you have an ulcer. She can detect an *H. pylori* infection and prescribe medication to heal it.

In the meantime, search your kitchen for these natural healers. Some may soothe your stomach, while others could shield it from a bacterial attack. And some might even be *H. pylori* exterminators.

If you can't give up spicy foods, don't. Show your doctor a list of your favorites and ask for a trial-and-error eating plan to determine which foods, if any, inflame your ulcer.

Cabbage. This member of the brassica plant family has long been a folk remedy for ulcers, and a recent study finally showed why. It's loaded with vitamins and plant compounds called phytochemicals, which protect your stomach's lining.

Broccoli, broccoli sprouts, kohlrabi, brussels sprouts, and cauli-flower — all members of cabbage's family tree — could be beneficial, too.

Cranberry juice. Health experts have known for years that cranberry juice fights urinary tract infections. This tart drink has its own type of phytochemicals that prevent bacteria from setting up shop.

Now researchers believe it might work against *H. pylori* in your stomach. One glass of cranberry juice a day could be enough to flush the bacteria out of your stomach — before they can dig in and wreak havoc.

Garlic. Next time you cook your favorite Italian dish, add plenty of this potent bacteria killer. In laboratory experiments, garlic extracts appeared to slow the growth of four different kinds of *H. pylori.*

Green tea. Reach for green tea when you're craving a warm drink and a little caffeine. Unlike black tea or coffee, green tea is gentler on your stomach. And drinking it regularly might help ease stomach inflammation.

Bees brew another stomach saver called propolis. This "mortar," which bees use for building hives, wiped out *H. pylori* in laboratory tests. More research is needed to see if it works for people.

Honey. Healers have used this golden delight for eons to fight infections. So it's no surprise today when scientists declare honey an ulcer healer. To help kill *H. pylori,* spread a tablespoon of honey on some bread and eat it an hour before meals and at bedtime. Don't drink anything with it so the honey will stay in your stomach long enough to work its healing magic.

Experts once believed only a special kind of New Zealand honey, called Manuka honey, had this special power.

But according to the latest findings, any unprocessed honey does the trick. Look for it at grocery stores or farmers' markets.

Sweet potato. The spud's tastier and more colorful cousin packs a two-fisted punch against ulcers.

Sweet potatoes are a great source of beta carotene, an antioxidant your body uses to make vitamin A. This vitamin protects your stomach lining and helps your stomach grow new cells.

And that's not all. Sweet potatoes are filled with fiber. Besides being a regular hero of your digestive system, fiber is especially protective in your stomach where it helps rebuild the lining.

Milk. Like cranberry juice, milk seems to flush bacteria from your stomach before they can cause problems.

Plus, it's a great source of vitamin A, which protects your stomach from ulcer-causing invaders.

Yogurt. This dairy snack is a veritable bacterial zoo. As dangerous as this sounds, the "bugs" in yogurt are really the good kind that battle the bad kind, like *H. pylori.*

What's more, yogurt can soothe your stomach when you take antibiotics to kill *H. pylori.*

When you feel that dull, gnawing pain coming on, reach for some yogurt. For best results, check the yogurt's label and make sure it says "active cultures." That means the good bacteria are inside, alive and kicking.

All of these foods can help your stomach when it's battling *H. pylori.* In some cases, however, there could be another explanation for your ulcer, such as nonsteroidal anti-inflammatory drugs (NSAIDs) or tumors. See your doctor to find the cause of your discomfort.

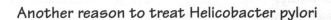

Another reason to treat Helicobacter pylori

You may have a vitamin B12 deficiency if you're infected with *H. pylori*. That's because this bacteria can interfere with how your body absorbs the nutrient.

In a study of 138 people with vitamin B12 deficiency, researchers found that more than half had *H. pylori*. When these people received medication that killed the bacteria, the deficiency vanished, too. This isn't surefire proof the bacteria interferes with vitamin B12 absorption, but it does suggest a strong link.

Here's how you can protect yourself:

◆ Bolster your diet with natural vitamin B12 sources, like tuna fish, clams, cottage cheese, beef, and chicken.

◆ Eat fortified cereals regularly. Tops on the list are General Mills Total, Kellogg's Special K, and Kellogg's All-Bran. All have 6 micrograms per serving, which is more than twice the daily recommended amount.

◆ Get tested for *H. pylori*. Your doctor will prescribe antibiotics if you're infected.

Left untreated, a vitamin B12 deficiency can lead to anemia, depression, nerve damage, muscle damage, and sometimes even paralysis.

Soothe your tummy with herbs

Herbal remedies have been popular for thousands of years, and now researchers know why. Herbs are great sources of powerful flavonoids and other antioxidants, compounds that sweep free radicals out of your body.

You probably already heard how free radicals can cause cancer, heart disease, and many other diseases. Now experts believe these rogue molecules may also have a role in forming ulcers.

"They may be a side effect of the inflammatory process," says Dr. Judith J. Petry, Medical Director of the Vermont Healing Tools Project. Free radicals are like pollution left behind when *Helicobacter pylori* bacteria attack your stomach. Then these scavenging free radicals irritate an already irritated ulcer.

By taking care of these free radicals, antioxidants may help heal your ulcer.

"The antioxidant properties of botanicals as well as pharmaceuticals," Petry agrees, "are believed to contribute to their anti-ulcer effects."

Here's a short list of botanicals, or traditional herbal remedies, that are full of ulcer-fighting antioxidants.

Licorice. It's more than just candy. Licorice aids your stomach by battling free radicals, protecting the stomach lining, stopping *H. pylori* from spreading, and easing inflammation.

Your best bet is to buy supplements of deglycyrrhizinated licorice (DGL). They appear to offer all the benefits of licorice without the side effects. Herbalists recommend taking two to four chewable 380-milligram tablets, 20 to 30 minutes before meals for two to four weeks.

Angelica root. Besides protecting you with antioxidants, this herb also seems to reduce stomach acidity and rejuvenate the stomach lining. You can buy supplements at health food stores. Just be sure to follow the dosage instructions, and avoid using this herb if you are taking blood thinners, like warfarin.

Caraway. Herbal experts know this tasty plant as a stomachic, which means a medicine that stimulates the actions of the stomach. To make a therapeutic tea, crush one to two teaspoonfuls of caraway seeds. Then pour about two-thirds of a cup of hot water over them. Drain after 10 to 15 minutes.

Lemon balm. This fragrant herb not only makes a delicious, soothing tea, it's a traditional remedy for stomach complaints and a potent bacteria killer.

To make a warm bedtime drink, pour a cup of hot water over half an ounce of the herb. Strain after 10 minutes.

German chamomile. This flower is the latest fad in herbal medicine, and it lives up to its hype.

It seems to reduce inflammation, fight bacterial infections, and boost your immune system. That's a great combination when you're fighting off an *H. pylori* infection.

To make chamomile tea, pour about two-thirds of a cup of boiling water over three teaspoons of the dried flower. Let it steep for five to 10 minutes before straining.

Bromelain. After analyzing the results of over 200 studies, researchers found this pineapple extract to be a possible ulcer blocker, as well as a first-rate anti-inflammatory and an excellent digestive aid.

You can find bromelain supplements at your local pharmacy or health food store. Follow the dosage instructions closely.

Just remember this important advice – see your doctor before self-treating an ulcer with herbs. "Ulcers can be fatal if inadequately treated," Petry cautions.

And since herbal supplements are not regulated in the United States, you could take bogus herbs and put yourself at risk without even knowing it. You really don't know if the product is what it says it is or not.

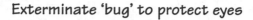

Exterminate 'bug' to protect eyes

Don't look now. *Helicobacter pylori* is at it again. This time the bacteria could attack your sight.

The stomach bug may have a role in glaucoma, the number two cause of blindness. In an eye-opening study from Greece, *H. pylori* infected nine out of 10 glaucoma sufferers. That's no coincidence.

Even more amazing, killing the bacteria with antibiotics appeared to reduce glaucoma symptoms and improve vision. Improvements are usually unheard of if you have this serious condition.

The researchers believe *H. pylori* can clog blood vessels in your eyes. This could cause eye pressure to build up, a major sign of glaucoma. If you treat the infection, the pressure seems to decrease.

Although more research needs to be done, the link looks promising. Exterminating *H. pylori* could be a cure for glaucoma, not just the symptoms. Keep your eyes peeled for the latest news.

Escape the menace of stomach cancer

Get rid of *Helicobacter pylori*, and you'll lower your risk of stomach cancer. Most people who get stomach cancer are infected with the bacteria. Yet, all hope is not lost, according to a Yale University study.

"Our results suggest," says researcher Susan Mayne, "that prevention strategies for these cancers should emphasize increased consumption of plant foods, decreased consumption of foods of animal origin with the possible exception of dairy products, and control of obesity."

So fill your plate with fruits, vegetables, whole grains, and legumes. The following foods are the most powerful stomach protectors around.

Broccoli sprouts. Some strains of *H. pylori* are strong enough to survive a battle with antibiotics. But they may not be able to escape from broccoli sprouts and their powerful disease-fighter, sulforaphane. In test-tube studies, this natural plant compound wiped out the toughest *H. pylori*.

"We showed that *Helicobacter pylori* strains resistant to multiple antibiotics were killed by sulforaphane in-vitro," reports Johns Hopkins researcher Jed W. Fahey.

This helpful substance also protects your stomach in other ways. "It boosts the body's own protective enzymes," Fahey explains, "which could have both cancer preventive and anti-oxidant benefits."

Though more testing needs to be done, it can't hurt to nibble on some broccoli sprouts. Or try these other brassica vegetables – broccoli, cabbage, cauliflower, and brussels sprouts. They also contain sulforaphane.

Black beans. An innovative new study showed folate may stop mutations from occurring in your genetic material, or DNA. Otherwise, these mutations could lead to cancerous cells. The study was just a start, since the researchers were only giving folate supplements to dogs.

But don't wait to enjoy foods high in this important B vitamin. Just two cups of black beans can give you a day's supply. Other good sources include dark leafy greens, asparagus, avocado, green peas, seeds, and enriched breads and cereals.

Tea. Men who regularly drank tea during a 12-year study seemed to have half the risk of stomach cancer as men who didn't drink tea. The reason could be powerful antioxidants called polyphenols.

"This study provides direct evidence that tea polyphenols may act as chemopreventive agents against gastric and esophageal cancer development," suggests one of the researchers, Mimi C. Yu. Green tea seems to have the most polyphenols, with oolong and black tea close seconds.

Strawberries. These mighty morsels are packed with vitamin C. Not only can this nutrient kill *H. pylori*, it's also an antioxidant that sweeps away the free radicals left in the bacteria's wake. Plus, strawberries are a low-acid source of vitamin C, so they won't irritate your ulcer. Broccoli, cantaloupe, peppers, and brussels sprouts share this claim to fame.

Guava. It's also important to have a low-acid source of lycopene, the famed antioxidant and cancer fighter. Guava is a winner, as are papaya and watermelon. Tomatoes and pink grapefruit are better known sources of lycopene, but their acidity could upset your stomach.

Spinach. Learn a lesson from Popeye and eat more spinach. In a Korean study, researchers discovered that eating spinach and cabbage reduced the risk of stomach cancer, while eating broiled meats and salty foods increased the risk.

Herbs and spices. If you need another reason to give up salty foods, look no farther than these flavorful mealtime additions. Basil, rosemary, turmeric, ginger, and parsley add zing to any dish, as well as a hefty load of flavonoids and other powerful antioxidants. Herbal experts say fresh herbs are much more potent than the dried variety.

Onions. Half an onion a day keeps stomach cancer away. That's what Dutch researchers discovered in a study of more than 120,000 men and women. Making half an onion part of your daily menu could cut your risk of stomach cancer in half. Onions contain quercetin and other antioxidants that can safeguard your stomach.

How to prevent a 'flare-up'

It's safe to smooch, according to the latest research. You can kiss your special someone without catching the dreaded *H. pylori* bacteria, experts say. But to prevent an ulcer flare-up, follow these tips.

◆ Eat fiber-rich and nutrient-packed foods, like fruits, vegetables, and whole grains.

◆ Space meals regularly throughout the day instead of just having snacks.

◆ Use caution with nonsteroidal anti-inflammatory drugs, also known as NSAIDs.

◆ Get a good night's sleep.

◆ Exercise regularly.

◆ Stop smoking.

◆ Learn to manage stress. Take up a new hobby or attend a yoga class.

◆ Practice moderation with stomach-irritating beverages, like coffee and alcohol.

Urinary incontinence

Tips to fix a leaky bladder

Over 200 million people have bladder control problems, and many of them find the situation so embarrassing they won't even mention it to their doctors. Women are more often affected than men, and the chances that you'll experience it increase with age.

If you're having problems controlling your bladder, tell your doctor. There are effective treatments available for urinary incontinence. In the meantime, here are some ways you can help yourself.

Check your menu. Many foods and drinks affect your ability to hold urine. Watch your intake of coffee, tea, carbonated drinks, citrus fruits, tomatoes, chocolate, sugar, honey, spicy foods, and milk products. It's quite possible one or more of these are adding to your problem.

Drink lots of water. Don't try to control your incontinence by drinking less. It is still important to keep your body well-hydrated. Experts recommend drinking six to eight glasses of water each day.

Take care of your skin. If your incontinence continues, the skin that comes in contact with urine may become irritated and infected. Keep your skin clean and dry by using mild soap, warm water, and soft towels. Ask your pharmacist to recommend a cream or ointment to help protect your skin.

Don't be ashamed to wear pads. You can wear an absorbent product to give you peace of mind and let you participate in activities you enjoy.

Train your bladder. By going to the bathroom on a strict schedule, you teach your bladder to hold more urine. Keep a chart or diary and begin by going to the toilet every 30 minutes. Gradually increase the time to every two to three hours.

Buy into biofeedback. A professional can train you in this technique to help you become more aware of how your body works. This will help you gain more control over your bladder.

Stay active. Exercising regularly will contribute to your overall health and keep your bowel movements regular. Constipation can affect incontinence.

Stop smoking. Tobacco smoke affects your bladder and urethra. And that hacking smoker's cough places a lot of stress on your bladder, which can lead to leakage. It's never too late to quit. Ask your doctor for help.

Work out. Kegel exercises are a great way to strengthen the muscles that control your urine flow. Sit comfortably with your legs uncrossed and your abdominal, thigh, and buttocks muscles relaxed. Then pretend you are trying to stop urinating. Keep these muscles tense for about 10 seconds, then relax. Repeat this tensing and relaxing 10 times, three times a day. Be patient. You may not see any improvement for at least six to eight weeks, and you may have to make the exercises part of your daily routine.

If you want to be sure you are doing them right, you can buy vaginal cones. Insert one of the weighted plastic cones into your vagina and tighten the muscles to hold the cone in place. If you are doing the Kegels correctly, the cone will not fall out. Remember to tighten these muscles before you cough, sneeze, or lift a heavy object to help control any leaking. Soon, you may not even have to think about it.

Urinary tract infection

Get on the right 'tract' to prevent UTIs

Visiting the bathroom is a routine part of every day. You probably don't give it a second thought – until it becomes painful. If you experience a burning, stinging feeling when you urinate, you may have a urinary tract infection (UTI).

Women are especially prone to urinary tract infections – one in five will have one sometime during her lifetime. Still, men over 50 can get UTIs from an enlarged prostate. Anything that interferes with urine flow causes urine to stay in the urinary tract longer. And bacteria have more time to get a grip and multiply.

Most urinary tract infections only cause temporary discomfort. If the infection spreads to your kidneys, however, it can cause permanent kidney damage or result in sometimes-fatal blood poisoning. Therefore, if you think you have a urinary tract infection, see your doctor right away – if you're right, he'll prescribe antibiotics.

Once you've had one urinary tract infection, you're likely to have more. Here are some natural nutritional strategies that may help prevent a painful infection in the future.

Cranberries. Modern medical research is beginning to confirm the healing powers of many home remedies, and that's certainly the case with cranberries. Studies show that cranberry juice really can prevent urinary tract infections. Some doctors think these tart little berries work by making your urine more acidic which slows the growth of bacteria. Other evidence suggests cranberries may work by keeping bacteria from clinging to your urinary tract.

To take advantage of cranberry's protective powers drink about 3 ounces of juice every day. One study found that the beneficial effects appeared only after four to eight weeks. So, for the most protection, drink cranberry juice regularly.

Vitamin C. Keep your refrigerator stocked with refreshing orange and grapefruit juice and you may keep UTIs at bay. Like the elements in cranberry juice, vitamin C and citric acid in citrus fruits may make your urine more acidic, thus making it more difficult for bacteria to grow.

Water. Ordinary water does an extraordinary job of washing bacteria out of your body before it has a chance to multiply. Drink at least six to eight glasses of water every day. Pale-colored urine is a good sign that you're getting enough. If your urine is dark, visit the water fountain a little more often.

Parsley. A green sprig of parsley on your plate doesn't just look good. It's a great source of vitamin C. What's more, it may act as a diuretic, which means it increases urine flow. And anything that increases the flow of urine could help reduce your chances of getting a urinary tract infection. So the next time a restaurant serves you a parsley garnish, don't just admire it – eat it for an extra bit of urinary protection.

Proven ways to beat bladder infections

Your doctor calls it cystitis. You may know it as a bladder infection. Whatever the name, once you've experienced the urgency, burning, tingling, and pain of a bladder infection, you don't ever want another one again.

Bladder infections, the most common type of urinary tract infections (UTIs), are the reason over 10 million women visit their doctors each year.

The bacteria that cause bladder infections, called *E. coli*, don't come from your urine because urine is sterile. That means it doesn't contain bacteria, viruses, or fungi. The bacteria get into your urethra, the tube urine travels through when it leaves your bladder, from your rectal area or skin. They travel up your urethra into your bladder, where they multiply, causing swelling, redness, and pain.

Most bladder infections can be prevented if you follow these six simple tips.

Don't fight the urge. Go to the bathroom whenever you feel the need, and empty your bladder completely each time. You may be tempted to resist the urge to urinate if you're too busy to bother, or you think it's going to be painful. Just remember – the longer urine sits in your bladder, the more likely it is to stagnate and allow bacteria to grow. Women should take special care to wipe from front to back. If you wipe from back to front, you may drag bacteria from your anus toward your urethra, giving germs an opportunity to set off an infection.

Urinate before and after sex. Emptying your bladder before and after sexual intercourse washes bacteria out of your urethra. It's also a good idea to wash your genital area before sex. This may help prevent spreading bacteria from one person to the other.

If you use a diaphragm or if your partner uses a condom with spermicidal foam, research shows you are more likely to get urinary tract infections. Consider other forms of birth control.

Take a shower instead of a bath. Baths may be relaxing, but sitting in a tub of water may give bacteria an opportunity to enter your urethra. Take showers instead whenever possible.

If your skin is sensitive, keep powders, soaps, creams, bath goods, or other hygiene products away from your genital area. Scented douches and feminine hygiene sprays may smell pretty, but they can also irritate your urethra.

Avoid foods that cause irritation. Certain foods and beverages may irritate your bladder. Common offenders include coffee, tea, alcohol, carbonated beverages, and spicy foods.

Stop smoking. In case you need another reason to ditch your cigarettes, smoking increases your risk for bladder infections.

Ask your doctor about new treatments. If you are postmenopausal, talk to your doctor about using a vaginal estrogen cream. It may help reduce the risk of urinary tract infections.

Varicose veins

Vanquish varicose veins naturally

Varicose veins are achy, painful, and even dangerous because of possible blood clots. But they're also ugly. The blue, swollen tangle of veins can transform your once fetching legs into unsightly road maps. If you want to keep your legs looking good without resorting to surgery, follow these helpful guidelines.

Change your diet. Load up on fiber and cut down on saturated fat, salt, and processed foods. Eat plenty of fruits, vegetables, and whole grains. This will help head off constipation, which contributes to varicose veins. In addition to fiber, fruits and vegetables also provide vitamins C and E, which help strengthen your circulatory system.

Exercise. Come up with a regular, moderate exercise routine. Walking, swimming, and yoga give your leg muscles a good workout, but be careful not to overdo it. "If someone has varicose veins and is killing themselves marathon running or becoming dehydrated, they're not doing any good," says George Nemecz, a biochemistry professor at Campbell University in North Carolina.

Lose weight. A combination of a healthy diet and a solid exercise program should help you shed those extra pounds, which pose an extra risk for varicose veins.

Wear comfortable clothing. Tight clothes, especially garments that fit too snugly around your waist, can obstruct your circulation. So can high heels. Opt for loose-fitting clothing and flats instead.

Don't stand still for long stretches of time. If you need to be on your feet, rock from one leg to the other or pace back and forth to keep your muscles moving.

Slip on support hose. These elastic stockings offer relief from your calves to your thighs. They come in handy if you must stand a lot for your job, if you're pregnant, or if you're overweight. Custom-made compression stockings can help in more severe cases. Put either type of stocking on early in the morning, before the blood gets a chance to pool in your lower legs.

Modify your bed. Raising the foot of your bed by about six inches helps keep the pressure off your veins at night. With your legs elevated, the blood should flow away from your aching calves. You can use wooden blocks or books to raise the foot of your bed.

Don't cross your legs when you sit down. This cuts off circulation. Instead, use a footstool to keep your feet level with, or even slightly higher than, your hips.

Soak in hot and cold water. Alternating between cold and hot water constricts and dilates your blood vessels. Your vessels get a workout and become stronger. Nemecz suggests keeping your legs in cold water for about 15 minutes and then switching to warm water for several minutes.

Stop smoking. This unhealthy habit narrows your blood vessels so blood has trouble moving through your body.

Know your family history. Thin skin, weak veins, and poor circulation might run in your family. If your mother had varicose veins, take precautions so you don't develop the condition, too.

Warts

Folksy ways to wipe out warts

The word "warts" may make you think of toads and witches, but they actually have nothing to do with either one. These pesky growths come from a virus and can appear on your hands, feet, or anywhere else the virus gets under your skin.

Warts generally are skin-colored and rough but can also be smooth, dark, and flat. They can even grow in instead of out if they're on the bottom of your foot. Those are known as plantar warts. It's important, therefore, to make sure you're dealing with a wart rather than another problem such as a corn, callus, or even a cancerous growth.

Since warts come from a virus, they will usually disappear by themselves once the virus has run its course. For this reason, many doctors will advise you to leave them alone. If you decide to remove them by traditional means, expect anything from blistering skin solutions to freezing chemical treatments to laser burning.

In many cases, though, home remedies may be just as effective. Though not scientifically proven, some folks swear these solutions work just as well as medical treatments.

Take your vitamins. All you need are a few vitamin tablets and some water to mix up these wart-dissolving remedies.

- Vitamins A and E are especially good for skin problems and can be applied directly to a wart. Simply break open a capsule, squeeze the liquid onto the wart, and rub it in once a day. It may take several months for the wart to disappear, so be persistent.

- Vitamin C is another effective wart fighter. Just crush up some tablets and mix with water to form a paste, and apply directly to the wart. Cover it with a bandage so the paste won't wear off. Vitamin C can irritate your skin so try to keep the mixture only on the wart.

Make these important vitamins part of your regular diet to help prevent warts in the first place. Also, make sure you get plenty of wart-busting nutrients such as beta carotene, zinc, sulfur, and B vitamins every day.

Check your medicine cabinet. Aspirin works just like vitamin C if you crush it and make a paste. The salicylic acid in this pain reliever will help dissolve the wart.

Play with your food. Some of the strangest wart cures come from things you eat. But they've had the most success of all, proving that folk wisdom and common sense often go hand in hand.

■ Bananas. They're probably not something you think of as a medical remedy, but even some doctors swear by the banana peel treatment. Dr. Matthew Midcap, an M.D. in West Virginia, has claimed a 100-percent cure rate in treating plantar warts with bananas, even in cases where all the traditional methods had failed. Simply cut a small piece of ripe banana peel and place it over the wart, white mushy side down. Tape the peel firmly in place and wear it all day. Change the peel each day after showering. The chemicals in the peel will soften and loosen the wart, eventually killing it.

■ Pineapples. While picking out your tropical fruit, don't overlook the pineapple. Pineapple juice is rich in a certain powerful enzyme that has proven an effective means of dissolving warts. Just soak a cotton ball in fresh pineapple juice, and apply it to the wart.

■ Potatoes. A raw potato slice contains similar chemicals for combating warts. Rub a slice on the wart several times a day.

Turn to your garden. A final self-treatment comes from your lawn or garden (although you may not be happy to find it there.)

Break open the stem of a dandelion, and apply the milky-white juice directly to the wart three times a day. After seven to 10 days, the wart should turn black and fall off.

As with any virus, successful treatment will depend on the state of your health and immune system as well as the virus itself. Don't give up if one method doesn't work for you – you can never tell what will cure your particular wart. But you may find that these folk remedies are just the thing to make your problem disappear.

Weight loss

Trick your body into losing weight

Do you turn to tricks and traps to lose weight? Weight-loss pills may sound like the answer to prayers, but these drugs can do more harm than good, not to mention costing you an arm and a leg. And single-food diets promising miracles can be nutritional nightmares. What you need are some healthy tricks that will melt those pounds off naturally and easily.

Lean on low-density foods. Here's a trick that will allow you to eat the same amount of food, feel just as full, but absorb fewer calories. The scientific fact behind this "magic" is food density – the amount of calories a food has per portion.

Low-density foods, like fruits and vegetables, are bulky and filling, but they don't carry a lot of calories. High-density foods, on the other hand, have a ton of calories crammed into small servings, mainly because they are loaded with fats and sugars.

To see the difference, try substituting the same amount of a low-density food for a high-density food – say 3 ounces of strawberries for 3 ounces of potato chips. You'll find you feel just as satisfied with the fruit, probably even more so. On top of that, you'll have saved yourself hundreds of calories.

Your goal is to eat more low-density foods such as produce, whole grains, and legumes, and cut down on fatty, sugary foods. But remember – even low-fat or fat-free snacks can be high-density because of their tremendous sugar content.

Fluff up your food. You may remember adding fluff to your peanut butter sandwiches as a child. That sugary confection will not help you lose weight, but food with extra air whipped in just might.

A study at Pennsylvania State University found these "fluffy" foods could help you eat less.

In the study, 28 men drank one of three different kinds of milkshakes before lunch. All three milkshakes had the same ingredients, but some were blended longer to add air and volume.

The men who drank the "airy" shakes ate 12 percent fewer calories at lunch. And they did not make up for it by eating more at dinner, meaning they kept those calories off.

So if you must snack, trick your taste buds by filling up on an air-filled treat, like low-fat frozen yogurt or butter-free popcorn.

Shrink your serving sizes. Cleaning your plate could be one of the only bad habits your mom taught you. Especially if you eat at a typical restaurant with a mountain of food on your platter. According to a recent study, the more you have on your plate, the more you'll eat. Fortunately, the opposite is true as well.

Weight loss comes down to one simple idea — you must burn more calories than you take in. Follow this advice and you may not have to worry about being over-weight again.

This is, essentially, a "Nothing Forbidden" diet plan anybody can follow. What it means is, you can have that slice of cheesecake but you have to burn those extra calories off or your body stores them as fat.

One great way to limit your serving size is to cook at home, where you can control how much food you cook. You also can try eating off a smaller plate to reduce the size of your portions.

Things get trickier when you eat out, but there are ways around a restaurant's generosity. Overcome huge entrées by splitting them with your spouse or friend. If you go it alone, put half your dinner into a doggie bag before you even start eating. That way, you won't be tempted by a full plate.

Limit food variety. A wide selection of food may be appealing when you're at a buffet, but it won't be when you get on the scale afterward. An overload of food appears to make your stomach's fuel gauge shut down. You're more likely to go beyond "full" just so you can taste everything. Experts think this tendency comes from our ancestors, who had to eat a variety of foods to guarantee they got all their nutrients.

The trick is to limit your snack selection. Store only one brand of chips in your cupboard or one type of cake in your fridge. You'll end up snacking less often because you'll get tired of the same old taste. On the other hand, stockpile a wide selection of fruits and vegetables. Variety in this case means getting a mix of nutrients that would make your ancestors envious.

Ditch high-calorie drinks. You've heard of a beer belly, but how about a soda belly? Experts say you can put on pounds without realizing it by drinking high-calorie beverages. Your body doesn't seem to register the drinks because they go right through you. So you take in hundreds of empty calories, and your stomach is still hungry for more.

Do yourself a favor, and replace most of your high-calorie drinks with low- or no-calorie ones like tea and water. You'll quench your thirst and save some pounds.

Green tea: Drink up and slim down

As if green tea weren't busy enough saving the world from diseases like cancer and heart disease, this popular drink can also help you lose weight.

In several tests, researchers gave a group of people green tea extracts — equal to between three and five cups of tea — at each meal. Their metabolism increased even more than the group taking caffeine pills.

This is great news for dieters since a higher metabolism means you burn calories faster. What's more, green tea can help you lose excess water weight – the kind that makes you feel bloated.

Just think, sipping tea for good health might also help you fit back into your skinny clothes.

7 ways fiber helps you win at losing

You've tried the hot dog diet, the banana diet, and the grapefruit diet. You've gone through diet pills, sweat suits, and supplements. Your home is littered with exercise equipment and videos that promised to help you lose extra pounds. But despite your best efforts, you can't seem to lose weight. What are you doing wrong?

Chances are, you're not eating enough fiber. Studies show obesity rates are tied to the amount of fiber people eat. In places like Kenya and Uganda, where they eat as much as 60 to 80 grams of fiber daily, less than 15 percent of the population are overweight. But the measly 15 grams a day eaten in more modern societies like the United States have contributed to the obesity of nearly 60 percent of adults. If you're one of them, you'll need to change your diet to include more fruits and vegetables because most fiber comes from plants.

You'll find it in whole-grain foods, legumes, leafy vegetables, fruits, nuts, root vegetables and their skins, and bran flakes. Besides allowing you more food on your plate, this important diet aid works on several levels to keep you trim.

Offers more food per calorie. One of the best things about fiber is that some of its calories don't count. That's because much of dietary fiber can't be digested. But fiber still fills you up. Experts say eating a diet high in fiber can trick your stomach into feeling full with fewer calories than you would normally eat.

Talk about "remote" control. The average person eats eight times more food while watching prime time television than at any other time.

Tune into breakfast instead. The body's ability to burn calories is greater in the morning than in the afternoon or evening.

Adults who eat breakfast every day tend to weigh less and have lower cholesterol.

Prolongs your meal. Most people would agree that the pleasure of food lies in the eating. A high-fiber diet requires lots of chewing and swallowing, and it can take a good while to finish a meal. Unlike many diets that limit food, you won't have to give up the joy of eating when you add fiber to your diet. It might actually take you longer than usual to polish off a lower-calorie meal.

Bulks up in your stomach. Ever finish a small meal while dieting and still feel hunger pangs? That won't happen if you eat more fiber. Water-soluble fiber absorbs water from your stomach and forms a kind of gel that swells up. Nerve receptors in your stomach signal your brain that your stomach is full, and you no longer need to eat. By filling up on fiber, you can go about your business without constantly feeling hungry.

Keeps you satisfied longer. But that's not all fiber can do. The thick gel it forms slows down the movement of food out of your stomach, so you end up processing your food more slowly. Instead of a high-calorie blast of energy that is quickly followed by tiredness and hunger, your energy supply is spread out over time.

Stabilizes blood sugar. Experts say this process affects your blood sugar in a healthy way. When you eat dried beans, barley, whole wheat, or pumpernickel bread, these foods slowly release their sugars for energy. Instead of your body getting surges of sugar from food, it gets its energy in steady amounts, which helps control insulin levels. In addition, a high-fiber meal can affect your blood sugar's response to the next meal you eat, keeping your blood sugar more stable throughout the day.

Boosts your hormones. You may not know it, but you have hormones working in your gastrointestinal tract. One in particular, called GLP-1, slows down the digestion process and gives you a sense of fullness. It can also help you lose weight. Studies on animals showed that eating fermentable fiber – the kind in fruits and vegetables – boosted their levels of GLP-1.

Blocks some calories. Dietary fiber can block the absorption of some of the fat and protein you eat. If you're overweight, that could be a good thing. One study showed that a group of people fed a diet containing only 20 grams of fiber a day absorbed 8 percent more calories than a group given 48 grams of fiber a day. For a typical 2,500-calorie diet, that's a difference of about 200 calories a day.

Just changing your fiber intake – without altering the number of calories you eat – could mean losing a couple of pounds a month. But be careful to add fiber to your diet slowly. Too much too soon can cause uncomfortable gas and bloating.

Get lean with beans

Lose weight without even trying. Just make beans a part of your diet – the part usually reserved for fatty meat.

Beans fill you up without lots of calories – only 225 calories in a one-cup serving. A study of healthy men showed that when they ate about two and a half cups of beans each day they ate significantly less fat and lowered their total cholesterol levels.

Another study found that the more canned beans men with high cholesterol ate, the lower their cholesterol. And even though the men were eating as many calories as usual, they lost weight.

But the heart-smart work of beans doesn't stop there. The fiber in legumes is like a bouncer for some big, bad cholesterol particles. Some of these thugs get shown to the door before they can do any damage to your arteries or heart.

Change dangerous flab to tight, flat abs

A "spare tire" around your waistline is a definite problem. Unwanted fat, especially at your midsection, increases your risk of heart disease, high blood pressure, diabetes, and some cancers. A recent study finds it can lead to lung problems as well. Naturally, you want to do something about it, but are gut-wrenching sit-ups the best way to get rid of a fat belly?

Not according to Dr. Bryant Stamford, a professor of physiology at the University of Louisville, Kentucky. Writing in *The Physician And Sportsmedicine*, he points out there is no such thing as spot reduction. When you exercise, you don't necessarily burn fat from around the muscles you are using. If you want to get the most out of your abdominal workout, follow these tips.

Choose exercise that burns the most calories. The fat you burn when you exercise may come from anywhere on your body, so Stamford recommends doing the activities that use the most calories. He says you'd have to do hundreds of sit-ups to equal the calories you'd burn on a brisk walk or jog.

Relax to stay trim. Exercise may be necessary for removing your potbelly, but reducing stress can help keep it off. For some reason, stress releases chemicals that cause fat to shift from other parts of your body to your waistline. Listening to music, talking things over with a friend or counselor, meditating, or doing yoga can help relieve stress. These practices also help you keep a positive attitude, which makes it easier to stick to your diet and exercise plan.

Tighten muscles for a sharper shape. Suck in your stomach when exercising, because a bouncing belly weakens the abdominal muscles. And don't forget to stretch your hamstrings. Strengthening these muscles on the back of your thighs helps prevent a swayback, which can make your stomach stick out even more.

Although they won't remove the fat, sit-ups can strengthen your abs, which protects your back as well. If full sit-ups seem too difficult, do just the second half, where you lower yourself down. Here's how:

■ Starting from a sitting position with hands at your sides, place your feet flat on the floor with your legs at a 90-degree angle. This way your abdominal muscles, not your legs and hips, will do the work.

■ Tense your belly and slowly – so your muscles work against gravity's downward pull – lower yourself until your back touches the floor.

■ Push yourself back up with your arms.

Repeat five times at first, adding a few more each time you work out. To exercise your abdominal muscles a little harder, increase resistance by crossing your arms over your chest.

A NEAT way to lose weight

If you drive your friends crazy by fidgeting all the time, now you have a good excuse – you're trying to lose weight.

Researchers had 16 people overeat for two months so they could measure what happened to those excess calories. Would they be stored as excess fat or burned off?

They found that the biggest factor in predicting weight gain among the overeaters was what they called the NEAT (non-exercise activity thermogenesis) factor. This was how often during the day a person changed positions, moved around, stretched, tapped their toes – in other words, fidgeted.

All the overeaters in the study gained weight, but that gain ranged from 2 pounds to 16 pounds with the more restless subjects gaining the least. Researchers speculate that the NEAT factor kicks in on some people when they overeat to compensate for the extra calories, while others just sit still and let the fat take over.

So if you've eaten a little more than you should, just tap your toes, drum your fingers, and fidget those extra calories away.

Fruit juice — a dieter's secret weapon

Looking for a delicious, safe way to cut a few extra calories out of your diet? Try drinking a cold, refreshing glass of orange juice or other fruit juice before meals.

According to a Yale study, drinking a glass of fructose-rich fruit juice a half-hour to an hour before a meal may help you eat less and still feel full. The study gave overweight people either an aspartame-sweetened diet drink, a glucose-water solution, a fructose-water solution, or plain water before lunch. Fructose is the type of sugar that is found in fruits.

The men who drank the fructose drink ate nearly 300 fewer calories at lunch, and the women who drank the fructose drink ate an average of 431 fewer calories, compared to people who drank plain water. The drink itself contained about 200 calories, which means each person saved between 100 to 231 calories. At three meals a day, that could save you at least 2,100 calories a week!

If you stirred a little pectin into your orange juice, you might be able to cut out even more calories. Pectin is a complex carbohydrate, made from certain ripe fruit, which is used to thicken jams and jellies.

One study found that people who drank a glass of orange juice with a small amount of pectin added felt fuller and ate less. Other studies have found that pectin can favorably affect blood sugar levels and cholesterol.

If you've resorted to over-the-counter or prescription appetite suppressants to help control your eating habits, it's nice to know that an occasional glass of tasty fruit juice before meals could be a healthy alternative.

Wounds and injuries

At-home first aid for minor wounds

Most cuts and scrapes get well without much attention. But some
wounds need more than a Band-Aid, but don't need a doctor's
attention. Here are a few tips:

Clean the wound. It's important to clean the wound to remove
any dirt or other foreign materials that might cause infection. Mild
soap and water are best. If the pressure of running water isn't
enough to remove all the dirt and debris, use a sterile pad to gently
brush the dirt out.

For easy cleaning of dirty wounds, keep a can of aerosolized saline
solution in your first-aid kit. You'll find it in the eye care section of
the pharmacy. Choose preservative-free saline for sensitive eyes
because it's safer for your wound.

Stop the bleeding. Many minor wounds stop bleeding on their
own. If it is still bleeding after you clean it, apply pressure to the
wound for a couple of minutes. If you can't easily stop the bleeding, you should see a doctor.

Kill the germs. You can help prevent infection in wounds by
applying antiseptic to kill the germs as soon as possible after the
wound occurs. You probably have a bottle of isopropyl alcohol or
hydrogen peroxide in the medicine cabinet. Both are excellent
antiseptics, but they may sting.

Iodine is also used as an antiseptic, but it burns and discolors the
surrounding skin. Iodine and hydrogen peroxide can be dangerous
if used on large areas. Decolorized iodine does not kill germs. If
you can't stand the sting, you can find nonstinging antiseptic ointments, creams and sprays at your pharmacy.

If you are really worried about infection, several antibiotic creams are available without a prescription. Apply a small amount (enough to cover your fingertip) one to three times a day. If your wound is too large to be covered by a fingertip's worth of antibiotic cream, you probably should see a doctor.

Cover the wound. Dressings are important for several reasons. They can be used to apply pressure to a wound to stop bleeding. Once the bleeding is stopped, they can absorb any fluid that oozes from the wound. They also help protect the wound from further damage and keep it clean.

Most minor wounds should be covered with a dressing that won't stick. First-aid kits usually contain this kind of dressing, which is readily available at any pharmacy. It's especially useful on hairy areas and on wounds that might tear easily. Wounds that drain may require additional absorbent dressing on top of the nonstick dressing. Don't put gauze directly on a wound because it might stick. Change the dressing daily, or more often if the wound is draining.

Secure the dressing. Use tape to firmly secure all four sides of the dressing. You can choose from several kinds of first-aid tapes. Cloth tapes won't cause allergic reactions, and they are very strong. Use cloth tape if the dressing is bulky.

Plastic tapes stretch with the skin, and the clear plastic lets you examine the wound without removing the tape. Paper tape isn't as sticky, so it doesn't irritate the skin as much as the other kinds. But it may come loose in areas where the skin moves. Don't use household tapes, like Scotch tape or masking tape, to secure a dressing.

Folk remedies for minor emergencies

When you're traveling, you never know what's going to hit you. Whether it's a bout of heartburn, a cold in ski season, or a sunburn at the beach, there's no substitute for being prepared. You could buy a prepackaged first-aid kit off the shelf of your local pharmacy, but if you assemble your own, you can combine safe commercial medications with folk remedies – all at a low cost. Here are some old-fashioned cures that are easy to take with you.

Baking soda. A little box of this miracle powder can do a lot. For starters, mix one-half teaspoon with one-half cup of water and drink it down for quick indigestion relief.

Banana peel or potato slice. When you can't find an ordinary bandage, these will take the "ouch" out of a nick or scrape. Just place the inside of a banana peel over your scratch, or tape a thin slice of raw potato to it.

Echinacea. Whether as a tea or supplement, this herb is your cold's worst enemy. It will ease the sniffling, sneezing, and achiness of wintertime woes in no time at all.

Ginger. For centuries, sailors have relied on ginger to keep them free of seasickness. For easy storage in your first-aid kit, try candied or crystallized ginger. An hour before you go on board, eat two chunks – each about one inch square by one-quarter inch thick. Then have one or two more every four hours as needed.

Panty hose and oats. To ease the itchiness of poison ivy, sunburn, or some other rash, cut off the foot of an old pair of panty hose. Fill it with rolled oats, tie the end, and hold the sack under the running faucet in your tub. Then settle down for a deep soak.

Rice and a sock. Fill an old sock with uncooked rice or birdseed and sew it closed. Either keep it in the freezer for a cold compress, or toss it in the microwave for hot relief. Make sure to place a cup of water in the microwave with it so the sock doesn't overheat and catch fire. This is great for sore muscles, migraines, or aching joints.

Rubbing alcohol. Fill a resealable plastic freezer bag with a mixture of water and rubbing alcohol and throw it in the freezer. For a softer, less frozen ice pack, add more alcohol.

Salt. Stir up one-fourth teaspoon of salt and one-half cup of warm water. Gargle and – presto – no more sore throat. Also, unstuff your stuffy nose, with a homemade saline nasal spray. Mix one-half teaspoon salt with eight ounces of warm water. Use either an empty nasal spray bottle or a bulb syringe.

Superglue. For faster healing of a paper cut or dry, cracked skin, drop on a bit of superglue. Just don't try this remedy on deep or bleeding cuts, and let the glue dry thoroughly before touching anything — especially your eyes.

Take-out condiments. A big ice pack won't work for tiny injuries. Instead, save up the individual packets of mustard and ketchup you can get at any fast-food joint. Keep them in the freezer, and they'll come in handy for little hurts.

Tea bags. If the sun left you well done, try dropping two or three tea bags into your bath. Or use moist gauze to hold them directly onto your burns.

Vinegar. For immediate relief from a sting or bite, dab vinegar on with a cotton ball.

Vitamin C. As soon as a nasty bug stings you, pop 1,000 to 1,500 milligrams of this wonder vitamin. It will act like a natural antihistamine to help soothe the sting and swelling.

White glue or tape. Lift out a splinter painlessly. Just dab on some white glue, let it dry, then peel the glue and the splinter right off. A piece of tape will work well on those tiny splinters that are hard to see.

Remember that pain, swelling, and other symptoms are your body's way of saying something is wrong. Pay attention and you'll recognize which everyday ailments and accidents you can treat yourself and which require professional help. Ear pain, toothaches, and vomiting, for instance, are more likely to need a doctor's call.

If you can't remember the last time you got a tetanus shot, even a minor cut or wound could require medical attention. Better yet, prevent tetanus by getting a booster every 10 years.

Bargain ways to beat bug bites

Don't spend a fortune on sprays and creams to soothe bug bites and stings. And don't expose yourself and your loved ones to harsh chemical bug repellents either. You can find a virtual pharmacy of natural alternatives at home – folk remedies that are tried-and-true ways to get quick relief.

Repel bugs naturally. The best way to relieve bug bites is to avoid them in the first place. A simple – and free – way to ward off mosquitoes, yellow jackets, and the like is to keep a few things in mind when you get dressed. Avoid wearing perfume or cologne, and leave your shiny jewelry indoors. These, along with bright colors and flowery-print clothing, attract bugs.

Nature also provides its own collection of bug fighters, which work just as well as any store-bought repellent. You can find the following fresh herbs and oils at your local grocery or health food store.

- Lavender. An essential oil made from this plant is great for warding off gnats and mosquitoes. Just mix two parts lavender oil with one part rubbing alcohol.

- Parsley, lemon balm, or basil. Rub the fresh leaves of any of these herbs on your skin if you want to stay welt-free.

- Garlic juice. People on the island of Sardinia douse themselves with this potent solution to keep away those dreaded bloodsuckers – mosquitoes, of course.

- Thyme. Ancient Greeks burned thyme to thwart stinging pests. Dried thyme keeps bugs out of your linen closet, too.

Find natural relief. If a creepy crawly still gets you, don't fret. Just try one of these homespun wonders. They might do away with the itch and irritation of a bite or sting.

- Aspirin. To swat the discomfort of bug bites, you don't have to swallow this over-the-counter drug. Put the aspirin right on your welt. First, make sure the stinger isn't still in your skin. (If it is, pull it out or scrape it away with a credit card or knife.) Then, just crush an aspirin tablet, wet it slightly, and bandage the sting. You can also use other nonsteroidal anti-inflammatories (NSAIDs), like ibuprofen. For even more relief, try dousing your bites with an antihistamine.

■ Basil. This herb is good for something besides topping tomatoes and mozzarella cheese. Crush fresh basil leaves and rub them on your bug bite for some sweet relief. You can keep the basil in place with a loose bandage.

■ Onions. Stop crying over that itching and swelling. Mash a fresh slice of onion and apply it, juices and all, to your sting. Onions contain phytochemicals, natural substances that will help reduce your swelling and pain.

■ Hot peppers. Just like an onion, these fiery remedies work wonders when you crush them and spread over your sting. A hot pepper won't lower the inflammation of a bug bite, but it will heat up your skin enough to take your mind off it. A few drops of hot sauce will do the trick, too. If your skin becomes too irritated, rinse the area immediately.

■ Peppermint and witch hazel. Peppermint oil can irritate your skin, so, like a hot pepper, a dab will make you forget your itchy bites. Witch hazel, on the other hand, can soothe and reduce swelling. That's why they make a perfect pair. Just mix two drops of peppermint essential oil for every ounce of witch hazel. Keep this precious potion in a cool, dark spot, and use a cotton ball to dab on as needed.

■ Baking soda and rubbing alcohol. Mix these two common household ingredients into a paste for quick and easy relief.

Test a small amount of any home remedy on the inside of your forearm, especially if you have allergies or sensitive skin. Don't use it if you develop redness or itching within 24 hours.

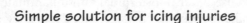

Simple solution for icing injuries

You know that icing a sprain, twist, bang, or other injury is a key step in good first aid. Ice lowers swelling and numbs the pain. But icing the old-fashioned way means sitting around and holding an ice pack to your injury.

Let plastic wrap do all that bothersome holding for you.

Just cut a roll of plastic wrap in half. Then take one side of it and use as much as it takes to secure the ice pack over your injury. The ice will stay in place while you're free to move around. You can even use plastic wrap to strap ice onto your back if that's where the pain is.

Don't let an injury keep you down. With this simple solution, you can stay moderately active while helping yourself heal.

Keep shinsplints at bay

Once you've made the decision to start exercising regularly, you don't need any barriers to stand in your way. You don't need your friends to encourage you to stay at home and chat, you don't need an impossible work schedule that leaves you no time for exercise, and you certainly don't need shinsplints.

Shinsplints can stop a successful exercise program in its tracks. The pain in the front of your lower leg can keep you from exercising, or even working, for several days, or longer if left untreated.

Ease into exercise. To avoid shinsplints, begin an exercise program slowly and carefully. Shinsplints are usually caused when you overuse and strain the muscles of your lower legs.

Be nice to yourself – don't do too much too soon. Even when your muscles are in good condition, you can overdo the exercise and end up with shinsplints.

Step out in style with shiny new shoes. Worn-out shoes are a common shinsplint culprit. Some people who run regularly believe the shock-absorbing power of running shoes wears out by about 300 miles.

Don't work out on hard surfaces. You should always do aerobics on a floor with a little give to it. Cement floors are too hard. And don't run on asphalt if you can avoid it.

Fix flat feet. Fallen arches can cause shinsplints. If you have flat feet, you may need shoe inserts. These will help get your legs correctly balanced.

Never push through the pain. If you start to feel pain in your lower legs while you are exercising, stop! If you keep going, you'll probably make the injury worse.

For the next three days, ice the area for 15 minutes twice a day. If the pain doesn't go away, apply moist heat for the next week. A hot shower or bath, along with gentle massage for five to 10 minutes, can help ease shinsplints.

When the shinsplints go away, you can begin exercise again. Start with half the workout you were doing before the shinsplints. Work up to your normal level over the next week or so.

Be sure to apply ice to the injured shin after you exercise, at least until the 10th day after the injury. (If you still have pain after 10 days, you should see a doctor.)

Stretch and strengthen. Lack of flexibility causes many shinsplints. Stretching should be a part of every workout. Stretching and strengthening exercises will also help heal your injury once you have shinsplints. Begin the exercises the third day after the injury.

Calf muscle stretch

■ Lean against a wall with your arms outstretched at shoulder height. Your palms should be flat against the wall.

■ Place one foot forward, keeping your back leg straight with the heel down.

■ Bend your front knee and push into the wall.

This should not cause pain, but you should feel tightness in the back of your calf. Hold the position for 10 seconds, then repeat with the other leg forward. Stretch each leg five to 10 times. Repeat two or three times a day.

Lower calf muscle and Achilles tendon stretch

■ Start in the same position as the previous stretch (with one foot forward).

■ Bend both knees and keep your heels on the floor.

You should feel tightness in the sides of your calf, but this should not be painful. Hold the position for 10 seconds, then stretch with the other leg forward. Stretch each leg five to 10 times. Repeat two or three times a day.

Calf raises (for strength)

■ Stand straight, holding onto something that will support you, like a table or chairback.

■ Rise up on your toes for five seconds.

Repeat 10 times, two or three times a day. If you don't feel pain, work your way up to 30 calf raises at a time.

As an alternative, you may want to ride a stationary bike for five to 10 minutes a day. Set the tension at low to medium. Work your way up to 20 minutes a day. Or you could try running in a pool to strengthen your calves.

3 ways to avoid bruising

When you got a bruise as a child, it was considered a badge of honor. As an adult, bruises can be ugly and even embarrassing. Thank goodness they usually aren't a serious problem. Most of them heal completely by themselves within a week or so. But if you are bruising a lot, even from bumps you hardly notice, you might have a vitamin deficiency.

Choose vitamin C. Every time you damage your body, you can break arteries, veins, and tiny capillaries. Blood seeps under your skin from these breaks and forms the familiar black and blue bruise. Vitamin C can strengthen your blood vessels by helping form collagen, a protein found in all your connective tissues, including skin. Even a minor deficiency of Vitamin C can make you bruise more easily.

To protect yourself from bruises, eat lots of fruits and vegetables rich in vitamin C, like oranges, strawberries, kiwi, papaya, red peppers, broccoli, and Brussels sprouts. And if you feast on these foods fresh and uncooked, you will get more of this important vitamin.

Stay OK with vitamin K. A bruise that seems to appear from nowhere or a cut that won't stop bleeding could be a sign of a vitamin K deficiency. You'll find this vitamin, which helps your blood clot, in spinach, cabbage, carrots, avocados, cucumbers, tomatoes, dairy products, and olive and canola oil. So fill your plate but, again, keep it fresh. Heating these foods doesn't seem to affect their amount of vitamin K, but freezing them may destroy it.

Examine your medication. If you take certain medications regularly, including aspirin, you just might bruise more easily – perhaps due to internal bleeding. See your doctor if you get a lot of bruises for no apparent reason or they don't heal within a few days. She may change your prescription or run some tests to rule out any serious disorders.

Wrinkles

Prevent wrinkles with yogurt

Going to the grocery store for a face lift? Not exactly. But you will find its shelves stocked with items that can either fast forward or turn back time.

Your skin is your body's largest organ, and so it's a huge target for free radicals. These unstable molecules form as you process oxygen. They travel throughout your body, damaging cells and causing all sorts of havoc – including wrinkles. You can't help producing free radicals, but you can help neutralize them.

Eat smart for smoother skin. Certain foods actually protect your face from wrinkles, according to Australian researcher, Dr. Mark L. Wahlqvist of Monash University in Melbourne. He found that if foods contain powerful antioxidants, in the form of vitamins, carotenoids, polyphenols, or other phytochemicals, they can counteract dangerous free radicals. Wahlqvist and his team of researchers learned these foods seem to fight wrinkles.

eggs	cherries
yogurt	grapes
spinach	melons
eggplant	prunes
asparagus	dried fruit
celery	apples
garlic	pears
onions	olives
nuts	jam

In addition, foods like olive oil contain monounsaturated fat, which resists skin cell damage.

It's easy to fit these into your weekly menu, and with so many to choose from, you can still enjoy a wide variety of dishes. Meals that blend vegetables, legumes, and olive oil – like those in a typical Greek diet – offer even more protection.

Avoid wrinkle-causing foods. Amid all the good news, researchers also discovered that certain foods have the opposite effect – they seem to encourage wrinkling. Saturated fat does not protect against sun damage and sugary products actually deteriorate your overall skin health.

milk (full-fat)	butter
margarine	ice cream
red meat	potatoes
soft drinks	cakes, pastries

Try to eliminate or cut back on these foods. Swap skim or fat-free milk for whole milk, water for soft drinks, fish for beef or pork, and fruit for sweet, sugary desserts. This just might be the recipe for a younger-looking you.

Yeast infection

Tips to soothe the savage yeast

Have you experienced the symptoms before — the annoying vaginal itch and thick, milky discharge? Was that first attack irritating, maybe even frightening? If you've suffered through just one yeast infection, you certainly don't ever want to go through it again.

But don't despair. While there is no permanent cure, there is good news. Here are the basic facts.

First-timers, see a doctor. You may have heard that itching and discharge signal the start of infection. But did you know that some women also experience soreness or rashes in the vaginal area, even pain during urination or intercourse?

And did you know that other, more serious conditions, like sexually transmitted diseases, can have some of the same symptoms?

Don't make the mistake of self-diagnosis when those first symptoms appear. You could be headed for trouble if you're treating the wrong disease. See your doctor. Remember, it often takes laboratory tests to know for sure.

Understand your risk. What are your chances for a yeast infection? To get some idea of what puts you at risk, you need to understand how and why a very small "yeast" can become so much trouble. At any given time, different areas of your body may be harboring colonies of *Candida*, the tiny fungus cells responsible for yeast infections.

Usually, that's no problem. When you're healthy, your body's various defense systems are quite capable of handling these little organisms. But when your immune system is weakened, fungus cells can quickly launch an invasion, especially in the genital tract, where there's plenty of warmth and moisture.

Stress, both mental and physical, hormonal changes from pregnancy or birth control, diabetes, common viruses and HIV are just some of the conditions that can put your immune system "out-of-order." Even the medication you took to cure another infection may be a problem. Some antibiotics are so strong they destroy both "good" and "bad" bacteria in your body. And you need those good bacteria because they are the first line of defense against fungal growth.

Keep your "cool." Sometimes you can't avoid the problems that leave your immune system vulnerable to infection. But you certainly don't need to make it easier for yeast to take hold. A yeast cell in your vaginal tract will thrive with extra heat and moisture. And unless you take a few precautions, you could be providing a very "warm welcome" for the next fungal invasion.

Blow it dry. Keep the area around your thighs and crotch as dry as possible. Take extra time to towel off after a shower, especially in the summer. You may want to use your blow dryer on a low setting to help dry your genital area after you bathe or shower. Change out of that damp bathing suit as soon as possible too. If you don't, you are inviting trouble.

Dress loose and cool. Try to avoid fabrics that keep moisture trapped against your skin. Summer or winter, the right clothes can make a healthy difference.

First, wear cotton panties. Second, don't wear pantyhose or tight clothes every day. Synthetic fibers in panty hose and underwear, even the heavy fibers in very tight-fitting jeans, won't draw dampness away from your body. Loose, cool, and dry – that's the prescription for smart dressing.

Wipe from front to back. Wiping front to back when you use the toilet will keep the bacteria in your rectum away from your vagina.

Don't douche. And don't use feminine hygiene sprays, deodorant sanitary pads or tampons, bubble bath, or colored or perfumed toilet paper. These products can change the acidic environment in your vagina, and that allows the yeast to grow.

Buy an over-the-counter anti-fungal medicine. Your best answer is medication that you apply after the symptoms appear. Inexpensive, nonprescription anti-fungal drugs usually destroy most yeast cells in just a few days. To make sure the infection is really cleared up, you should use the full supply of medicated inserts or suppositories as directed.

And always heed the drug manufacturer's warnings – if the symptoms don't improve within three days, be sure to see your doctor. Don't let the problem drag on. It could be a lot more serious than a yeast infection.

Ward off infections with food

If you're a woman, you're likely to have at least one yeast infection in your lifetime. Yeast infections are just one type of vaginitis, an inflammation of your vagina. You always have a small amount of yeast in this area, but when it multiples, it can cause itching, burning, and irritation.

Luckily, several key nutrients may help fight off the specific bacteria that cause these annoying infections.

Folic acid. This B vitamin protects you from vaginitis and may decrease your risk of cervical cancer as well. Researchers think low levels of folic acid may make it easier for cancer-causing substances to attack your tissues. So protect yourself by eating more cantaloupe, asparagus, beets, liver, and green, leafy vegetables like spinach and turnip greens. If possible, eat these fruits and vegetables raw since cooking destroys up to half of this important vitamin.

Iron. This mineral is especially important to a woman's health before menopause. Foods high in iron include shellfish, red meat, dried fruit, and spinach. Adding foods high in vitamin C will help your body absorb the iron better. For example, stir-fry some vitamin C-rich broccoli with your shrimp, or garnish your spinach salad with orange slices.

Magnesium. Research finds that women who have recurring yeast infections are likely to have low levels of magnesium. To make sure you get plenty of this mineral, eat nuts, whole grain foods, and dark green vegetables like spinach and broccoli.

Zinc. About half of all adult women in the United States get substantially less than the recommended daily amount of zinc. That's bad news for them because this mineral may help fight yeast infections. Foods rich in zinc include seafood, red meat, poultry, legumes, and whole grains.

Selenium. Scientists don't know how selenium fights vaginal infections, but they do know that women with chronic cases of vaginitis have low selenium levels. To get plenty of selenium, make sure you eat unprocessed foods like grains and fresh fruits and vegetables

Vitamin A. The lining of your vagina acts as a protective barrier against bacteria. If cells die, bacteria can invade and cause infection. Vitamin A keeps these cells alive and well so it's your first line of defense against vaginal infections. Foods rich in vitamin A include liver, fortified dairy products, and eggs. You can also eat foods high in beta carotene, which your body turns into vitamin A, such as spinach, sweet potatoes, carrots, and papaya.

Fatty acids. Inflammation often goes hand-in-hand with yeast infections. To fight it, you need to eat more of the essential fatty acids omega-3 and omega-6. Have some fish two or three times a week, along with small amounts of vegetable oils like canola, safflower, sunflower, or olive oil. Seeds, nuts, poultry, and eggs contain good amounts of fatty acids as well.

Yogurt. Eating a cup of yogurt every day may be an easy and delicious way to sidestep yeast infections. *Lactobacillus acidophilus* is a good kind of bacteria found in the vagina. Scientists believe it may fight off the bad bacteria that result in yeast infections. Many yogurts also contain *L. acidophilus* cultures. In several studies, researchers had women eat 8 ounces of bacteria-rich yogurt every day for several months. Most of the women had fewer vaginal infections during that time.

Multi-talented nutrients

Simply put – you can't live without vitamins and minerals. Your body needs a certain amount each day. Missing your daily quota once in a while won't hurt. But if you shortchange yourself on a regular basis, you put yourself in danger.

Luckily, you'll find plenty of vitamins and minerals in grains, legumes, fruits, seafood, lean meats, vegetables, and other healthy foods. Include these foods in your daily diet, and you'll protect yourself from many diseases, including cancer, heart disease, arthritis, cataracts, depression, anemia, macular degeneration, thyroid disease, and memory loss – just to name a few.

Vitamins. All vitamins are one of two types, fat-soluble or water-soluble. Although they are both equally important, they are used differently by your body.

Your body absorbs, transports, and stores fat-soluble vitamins with bile and fat. That explains their name. It also explains why you should avoid taking these vitamins in high doses, especially in supplement form. Fat-soluble vitamins naturally build up in your fatty tissues and liver, and their levels only go down gradually as your body uses them.

If you take in too much at once, your body has no way of dumping the excess. That can leave you very sick. Getting the fat-soluble vitamins – A, D, E, and K – from food sources is the best way to get the right amount.

In your body, water-soluble vitamins, which include the B vitamins and vitamin C, float freely in your blood or in the watery fluid between your cells. Yet, they don't stick around for long. Your body doesn't store them. Instead, it uses them or flushes them out through your kidneys.

This means you don't have to worry about overloading on water-soluble vitamins. But keep in mind you do need to replace them often. These nutrients generally help your body carry out its day-to-day chores, and each one has important jobs to do.

Some vitamins also act as antioxidants. They're your body's tiny foot soldiers, tirelessly watching over you and fighting off harmful molecules called free radicals. A free radical has one or more extra electrons that make it unstable, so it goes off and steals an electron from another molecule to make itself stable.

This causes a chain reaction that eventually results in tissue damage and disease. Antioxidant vitamins come to your rescue by giving up electrons to stabilize free radicals, which helps keep your body healthy.

Minerals. When you think of precious minerals, you probably think of gold and silver. But where your health is concerned, other minerals – like calcium and iron – are far more precious.

Each dietary mineral is unique and carries out its own special life-giving task. Scientists have divided these nutrients into two groups, major and trace minerals, depending on how much of the mineral is in your body.

If you could remove all the minerals in your body and place them on a scale, they would weigh about 5 pounds. Almost 4 pounds of that would be calcium and phosphorus, the two most common major minerals. The other major minerals – potassium, sulfur, sodium, chloride, and magnesium – would make up most of the remaining pound.

Trace minerals are small but powerful. Each one makes up only a tiny percentage of your total body weight, but their small amounts only make them more valuable. Iron, boron, manganese, copper, iodine, fluoride, molybdenum, selenium, zinc, and chromium are trace minerals.

Understand your daily requirements

RDA, DRI, IU, RE – these are all ways of measuring vitamins. It can be confusing if you don't know what these terms stand for. Get them straight to make sure your diet is vitamin-complete.

DRI (dietary reference intakes) are new guidelines that replace the RDA (recommended dietary allowances) you're probably familiar with.

The DRI include the RDA but also take into account new research on disease prevention, the upper limits you can safely take, and the average nutrients required by healthy people throughout the world.

The DRI are not minimum requirements, but rather they are recommendations for the best and safest amounts for people in each age group.

Experts believe the DRI more accurately show a person's daily nutrition requirements. To understand DRI recommendations, keep in mind that anything ending in "grams" is a metric weight.

Micrograms (mcg) are the smallest, and it takes 1,000 mcg to make 1 milligram (mg). Likewise, it takes 1,000 mg to add up to 1 gram.

Fat-soluble vitamins are sometimes listed as IUs (international units). And you may see RE (retinal equivalent) or RAE (retinal activity equivalent) used to measure vitamin A.

All of these measures can help you figure out how much of the vitamin you are getting. Just be sure your intake falls within the recommended guidelines.

Phytochemicals. Besides vitamins and minerals, other natural chemicals in plants, called phytochemicals or phytonutrients, can have a powerful effect on the human body. Found in fruits, vegetables, herbs, and spices, these tens of thousands of substances have been used to treat and prevent diseases since ancient times.

Many cultures, like the Chinese and American Indians, have always looked to plants for healing. And even today, the World Health Organization says about 80 percent of the people on earth use natural medicines, mostly involving plants.

Unfortunately, modern man's passion for science and advanced technology has inflated the market for pills and capsules, replacing whole sources of nutrition from foods. That's why you'll find a host of supplements in stores and on the Internet offering an easy supply of phytochemicals.

But there is very little evidence these plant chemicals do the same job once you take them out of their original "package," possibly because the chemicals need other parts of the plant to work properly. As always, the best way for you to get the most benefit from phytochemicals is to eat whole foods.

It's easy. Choose fruit for snacks and dessert, double the amount of vegetables you normally eat, season your dishes with herbs and spices, and plan several meatless meals that contain legumes and whole grains. In addition, cook your vegetables lightly since heat destroys many of these natural substances.

Some foods contain literally hundreds of phytochemicals and some specific phytochemicals do more than one kind of job. Carotenoids, flavonoids, isothiocyanates, phytosterols, and polyphenols are the most common types.

For more information about vitamins, minerals, and phytochemicals, be sure to check out the helpful charts that follow.

Fat-soluble vitamins

Vitamin	Dietary Reference Intakes* (DRI)		What it does	Good sources	Suggested daily servings
	Women (age 51+)	Men (age 51+)			
A (Retinol)	700 RE	900 RE	• controls eyesight • builds new cells • protects skin and mucous membranes • fights infection and free radicals	liver, dairy, eggs	1/3 oz. of beef liver or 6 cups of skim milk
D (Calciferol)	10–15 mcg or 400 IU	10–15 mcg or 400	• builds bones • controls calcium and phosphorus levels in your body	fortified milk, eggs, liver, sardines	4 cups of skim milk or 9 oz. of shrimp or 4 oz. of salmon
E (Tocopherol)	15 mg or 22 IU	15 mg or 22 IU	• fights free radicals	vegetable oils, dark leafy greens, nuts and seeds, wheat germ	2-1/2 oz. of wheat germ or 5 Tbs. of canola oil or 1 oz. of sunflower seeds
K (Phylloquinone)	90 mcg	120 mcg	• forms blood clots • controls calcium levels	dark leafy greens, cruciferous veggies	1/2 cup of broccoli or 1 cup of cabbage

Vitamin	Dietary Reference Intakes* (DRI)		What it does	Good sources	Suggested daily servings
	Women (age 51+)	Men (age 51+)			
			Water-soluble vitamins		
B1 (Thiamin)	1.1 mg	1.2 mg	• produces energy • sends nerve messages • brings on healthy appetite	whole grains, nuts, legumes, pork	2-1/2 cups of cooked black beans or green peas or 5 slices of watermelon
B2 (Riboflavin)	1.1 mg	1.3 mg	• produces energy • helps vision • builds new cells	dairy, dark leafy greens, whole grains	2 cups of skim milk or 2 cups of raisin bran
B3 (Niacin)	14 mg	16 mg	• produces energy • builds DNA	protein-rich foods, dairy foods, fish, nuts, whole grains	1 can (6 oz.) of light tuna or 4 oz. of chicken breast
Folate (Folic acid)	400 mcg	400 mcg	• makes and repairs DNA • removes homocysteine from blood	dark leafy greens, legumes, seeds, enriched breads and cereals	2 cups of cooked black beans or cooked frozen spinach or 1-1/4 cups of toasted wheat germ
B12 (Cobalamin)	2.4 mcg	2.4 mcg	• makes new cells (especially red blood cells) • protects nerves	meats, fish, dairy foods, eggs	2 cups of low-fat cottage cheese or 1-1/2 oz. of salmon

Vitamin	Dietary Reference Intakes* (DRI)		What it does	Good sources	Suggested daily servings
	Women (age 51+)	Men (age 51+)			
B6 (Pyridoxine)	1.5 mg	1.7 mg	• makes red blood cells • builds proteins • regulates blood sugar • makes brain chemicals • protects immune system	dark leafy greens, seafood, legumes, whole grains, fruits and veggies	3 bananas or 3 potatoes or 6 oz. of beef liver
Biotin	30 mcg	30 mcg	• produces energy • helps body use other B vitamins	liver, egg yolks, legumes, nuts, cauliflower	3 oz. of peanut butter or 3-1/2 oz. of oatmeal
B5 (Pantothenic acid)	5 mg	5 mg	• produces energy	whole grains, organ meats, broccoli, avocados	2 cups of wheat germ or 6 oz. of bran
C (Ascorbic acid)	75 mg	90 mg	• makes collagen for skeleton and skin • fights free radicals • bolsters immune system • helps body absorb iron	citrus fruits, dark leafy greens, cruciferous veggies, bright-colored fruits and veggies	1 cup of strawberries or raw broccoli or 1 orange or whole grapefruit

*DRI are new tools for figuring out how much of a vitamin or mineral you should include in your daily diet. They replace and add to the older RDA (recommended dietary allowances).

Mineral	Dietary Reference Intakes* (DRI)		What it does	Signs of deficiency	Good sources
	Women (age 51+)	Men (age 51+)			
			Major minerals		
Calcium	1,200 mg	1,200 mg	• builds bones and teeth • contracts muscles and nerves • sends nerve messages • controls blood pressure	bone loss (osteoporosis)	dairy foods, small bony fish, legumes
Chloride	750 mg	750 mg	• makes stomach juices for digestion • balances levels of other minerals	muscle cramps, trouble concentrating, loss of appetite	salt
Magnesium	320 mg	420 mg	• builds bones and teeth • relaxes muscles • makes proteins • helps body use nutrients • steadies heart rhythm	Tiredness, loss of appetite, muscle cramps and twitches, convulsions, depression, confusion	nuts, legumes, whole grains, dark leafy greens, seafood
Phosphorus	700 mg	700 mg	• builds new cells • produces energy	loss of appetite, tiredness, pain in bones	meats, dairy foods

Mineral	Dietary Reference Intakes* (DRI)		What it does	Signs of deficiency	Good sources
	Women (age 51+)	Men (age 51+)			
Potassium	3,500 mg	3,500 mg	• sends nerve messages • relaxes nerves • maintains chemical balances • steadies blood pressure	Dehydration, weakness, trouble concentrating	fresh fruits and vegetables, fish, legumes, dairy foods
Sodium	500 mg	500 mg	• balances fluid levels • sends nerve messages	muscle cramps, trouble concentrating, loss of appetite	salt, processed foods
Sulfur	Not determined	Not determined	• builds vitamins and proteins • removes toxic chemicals	protein deficiency	all protein-packed foods
Trace minerals					
Boron	Not determined	Not determined	• helps body use calcium • builds bones and joints	bone loss (osteoporosis), joint pain (osteoarthritis)	non-citrus fruits, nuts, legumes, dark leafy greens
Chromium	20 mcg	30 mcg	• produces energy • balances blood sugar level	high blood sugar level	whole grains, meats, nuts, cheese

Mineral	Dietary Reference Intakes* (DRI)		What it does	Signs of deficiency	Good sources
	Women (age 51+)	Men (age 51+)			
Copper	900 mcg	900 mcg	• makes red blood cells • produces energy • fights free radicals	Weakness, pale skin, unhealed wounds	organ meats, seafood, nuts, seeds
Fluoride	3 mg	4 mg	• protects bones and teeth	dental cavities	tea, seafood, tap water
Iodine	150 mcg	150 mcg	• makes thyroid hormones • steadies metabolism	goiter	seafood, salt, dairy foods
Iron	8 mg	8 mg	• carries oxygen throughout body • produces energy	Weakness, pale skin, trouble concentrating	meats, eggs, legumes, dried fruits
Manganese	1.8 mg	2.3 mg	• produces energy • builds bones and joints	None known	nuts, legumes, whole grains, tea
Molybdenum	45 mcg	45 mcg	• fights free radicals	severe headache, rapid heartbeat, confusion	dairy foods, legumes, whole grains
Selenium	55 mcg	55 mcg	• makes thyroid hormones • fights free radicals • strengthens immune system	muscle weakness and pain, cataracts, heart trouble	meats, seafood, whole grains

Mineral	Dietary Reference Intakes* (DRI)		What it does	Signs of deficiency	Good sources
	Women (age 51+)	Men (age 51+)			
Zinc	8 mg	11 mg	• produces energy • makes DNA • helps body use vitamin A • fights free radicals • heals wounds • boosts immune system	Diarrhea, infections, loss of appetite, weight loss, unhealed wounds	meats, shellfish, legumes, whole grains

*DRI are new tools for figuring out how much of a vitamin or mineral you should include in your daily diet. They replace and add to the older RDA (recommended dietary allowances).

Phytochemical	Type	Possible benefits	Good sources
Anthocyanins	Flavonoid	• acts as antioxidant to fight heart disease • protects vision • combats cancer	blueberries, strawberries, raspberries, blackberries, currants

Phytochemical	Type	Possible benefits	Good sources
Beta carotene	Carotenoid	• preserves eyesight • strengthens immune system • works as an antioxidant to fight heart disease, cancer, memory loss, rheumatoid arthritis, respiratory distress syndrome, liver disease, Parkinson's disease, and complications of diabetes	carrots, sweet potatoes, pumpkins, mango, cantaloupe, apricots, spinach, broccoli
Capsaicin		• regulates blood clotting	chili peppers
Catechin	Polyphenol	• protects against cancer • fights heart disease	green tea, red wine, red grape juice
Curcumin	Polyphenol	• protects against stomach, breast, lung, colon, and skin cancers • fights inflammation	turmeric, ginger
Daidzein	Flavonoid	• protects against breast, colon, ovarian, and prostate cancers • guards against osteoporosis	legumes, soybeans*
Ellagic acid	Polyphenol	• works as an antioxidant to fight cancerous tumors, especially of the lung, liver, skin, and esophagus	strawberries, grapefruit, blackberries, blueberries, raspberries, walnuts, pomegranates
Genistein	Phytosterol	• protects against breast, colon, ovarian, and prostate cancers • strengthens bones • fights menopause symptoms	soybeans*

Phytochemical	Type	Possible benefits	Good sources
Lignans	Phytosterol	• protects against breast, colon, ovarian, and prostate cancers • fights heart disease	whole grains, flaxseed
Limonene	Monoterpene	• protects against cancer	orange and lemon peel, cherries
Lutein	Carotenoid	• preserves eyesight • protects against cancer	collard greens, spinach, kale, broccoli, turnip greens, zucchini, corn, kiwi, red seedless grapes, egg yolks
Lycopene	Carotenoid	• protects against esophageal, stomach, and prostate cancers • preserves eyesight	guava, papaya, pink grapefruit, tomatoes, watermelon
Phytic acid		• protects against cancer and heart disease	wheat germ, soybeans*
Quercetin	Flavonoid	• fights inflammation • protects your arteries • fights allergies • protects against cancer • fights bacteria	tea, red onions, buckwheat, citrus fruits
Resveratrol	Flavonoid	• fights heart disease • protects against cancer • fights inflammation	red grapes, red wine

Phytochemical	Type	Possible benefits	Good sources
Sulforaphane	Isothiocyanate	• protects against cancer	broccoli, cabbage, kale, cauliflower, brussels sprouts, ginger, onions, bok choy
Tannins		• protects against cancer	tea, whole-grain cereals
Zeaxanthin	Carotenoid	• preserves eyesight	broccoli, grapes, spinach, collard greens, kale, turnip greens, zucchini, orange peppers, kiwi, red seedless grapes, egg yolks

*Warning: New research claims that soy may accelerate brain aging.

Index

A

Acetaminophen, asthma and 31
Acne 1–5
Acupressure, for sinusitis 274
Acupuncture 267
Alcohol
  bladder infection and 315
  breast cancer and 45
  cataracts and 74
  dry mouth and 125
  gout and 143
  heart disease and 170
  heartburn and 161
  impotence and 200
  insomnia and 205
  kidney stones and 215
  macular degeneration and 220
  memory loss and 223
  motion sickness and 235
  psoriasis and 258
  rosacea and 270
  stroke and 288
  ulcers and 310
  warfarin and 291
Allergies 6–10
Aloe vera
  for psoriasis 257
  for skin rash 8
Alzheimer's disease 11–18
  See also Memory loss
Amino acids, for chronic
    fatigue 79
Anemia 19–21
Angelica root, for ulcers 305
Antihistamines, sinusitis and 273
Antioxidants
  for Alzheimer's 12

for cancer 55
for memory 222
for rheumatoid arthritis 265
for stomach cancer 308–310
for ulcers 304–306
for wrinkles 342
Anxiety 22–28
  See also Stress
Apple juice
  for gallstones 140
  kidney stones and 215
Apples, for diarrhea 116
Apricots 60
Aromatherapy
  for depression 102
  for stress 25
Arthritis
  tips for 241
  See also Osteoarthritis,
      Rheumatoid arthritis
Artichokes, for high
        cholesterol 196
Aspirin
  cataracts and 73
  for Alzheimer's 14
  for bug bites 336
  for colon cancer 89
  for diabetes 111
  for warts 320
  gout and 142
  stroke and 289
Asthma 29–33
Atherosclerosis
  impotence and 198
  memory loss and 225
  See also Heart disease
Athlete's foot 34–35

B

C

D

M

N

O

Wounds 332–341
Wrinkles 342

X

Xanax, for tinnitus 294

Y

Yeast infection 344–348
Yoga
  for fibromyalgia 135
  for tinnitus 295
Yogurt
  for acne 3
  for bad breath 40
  for canker sores 61
  for celiac disease 78
  for indigestion 159
  for ulcers 303
  for yeast infection 347

Z

Zeaxanthin, for macular
      degeneration 219
Zinc
  for canker sores 64
  for ears 232
  for immune system 83
  for macular degeneration 219
  for prostate 253
  for sinusitis 275
  for yeast infection 347